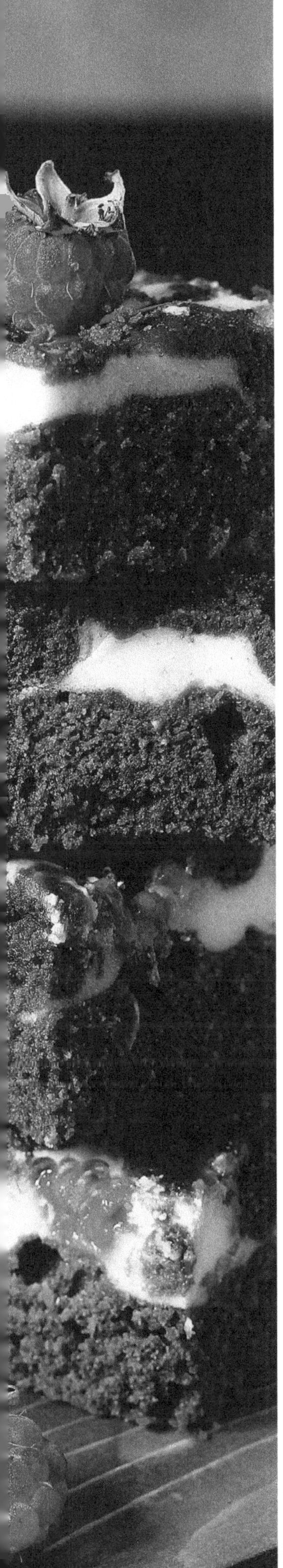

The Complete Acid Reflux Solution Cookbook

Delicious Recipes and Easy Meal Plans for GERD and LPR Relief. Your Simple Diet Plan for Heartburn-Free Days

By
Sarah Combs

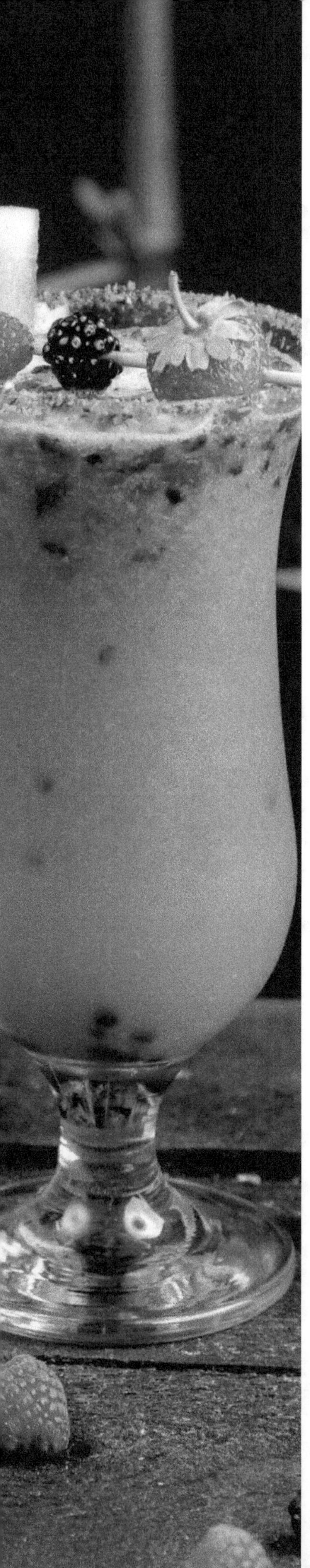

Copyright Warning

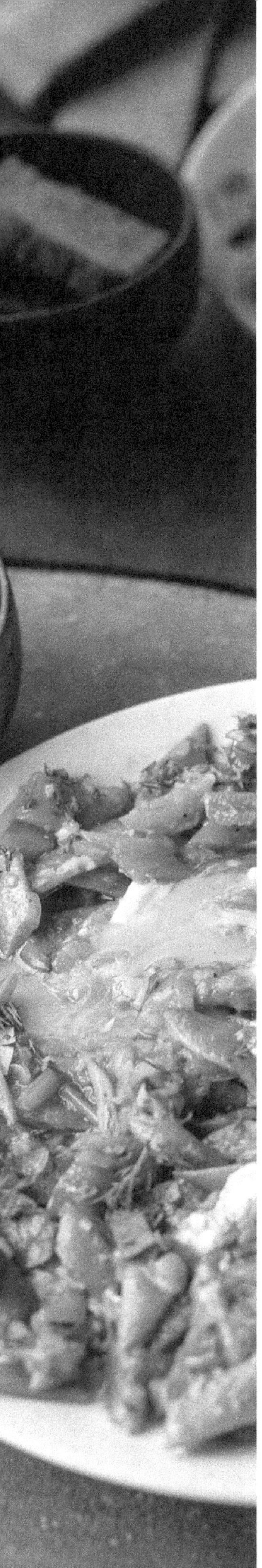

Table of Contents

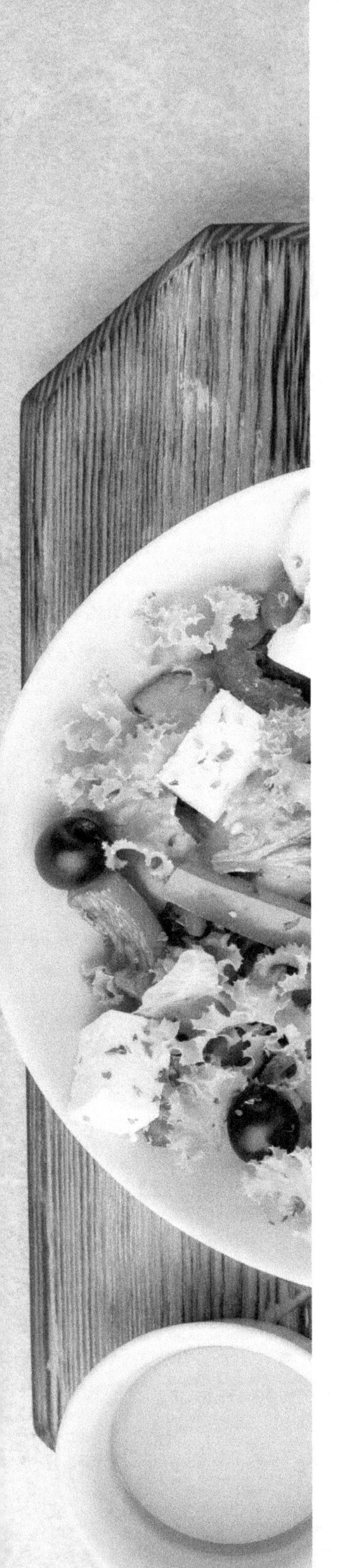

Introduction

Welcome to "The Complete Acid Reflux Solution Cookbook," your guide to navigating the turbulent waters of acid reflux with delectable and relaxing meals. If you've ever felt a burning sensation rise up your chest after a meal or if you've avoided specific foods for fear of causing discomfort, you're not alone. Acid reflux, also known as heartburn, is a common digestive condition that affects millions of people worldwide. But what is acid reflux, and why does it occur? Imagine your stomach as a bustling kitchen, working hard to digest the food you've eaten. Normally, a muscular valve called the lower esophageal sphincter (LES) works as a gatekeeper, keeping stomach contents where they should be. However, sometimes that gate fails to close properly, enabling stomach acid to wash back up into the esophagus. This acidic rush can cause the typical burning feeling as well as other painful symptoms such as regurgitation, bloating, and chest pain.

So, what is the source of this failing gate? Yes, it might be a mix of reasons. Certain meals and beverages, such as spicy dishes, citrus fruits, and caffeine, are known to cause reflux symptoms. Lifestyle habits such as overeating, eating too close to bedtime, and lying down after meals might aggravate the problem. And don't forget about stress, which may wreak havoc on our digestive system and exacerbate reflux symptoms. But do not worry, my reader, for this is where "The Complete Acid Reflux Solution Cookbook" comes in. Throughout this book, we'll look at the causes and symptoms of acid reflux, as well as how you can use food to control your digestive health. No more boring diets or restrictive eating—our objective is to provide you with the knowledge and skills you need to consume great meals without fear of discomfort.

So, whether you're a long-time reflux sufferer or just starting to experience the occasional flare-up, consider this book your road map to relief. We'll go on a journey to digestive wellness, one delicious recipe at a time. Prepare to bid heartburn farewell and welcome to a happier, more comfortable you. Welcome to "The Complete Acid Reflux Solution Cookbook."

Chapter 1

The Basics of Acid Reflux: Unraveling the Mystery Within

Welcome to the first step on your path to digestive health: learning about acid reflux, a disorder that affects millions of people worldwide. In this chapter, we'll go on a journey of discovery, peeling back the layers of complexity to unveil the underlying workings of this prevalent but frequently misunderstood illness.

Acid reflux is a digestive system problem that causes stomach acid to flow backward into the esophagus. This condition, known as gastroesophageal reflux, occurs when the lower esophageal sphincter, a muscle valve that typically stops stomach contents from regurgitating into the esophagus, fails to function correctly. What was the result? Acidic stomach acids wreak havoc on fragile esophageal tissues, causing a cascade of discomfort ranging from slight irritation to severe agony. But what causes this disruptive flood of acid? While the exact causes differ from person to person, some common triggers have been shown to worsen reflux symptoms. These include dietary elements like spicy or acidic foods, fatty meals, and caffeine-containing beverages, as well as lifestyle habits like smoking, binge drinking, and lying down after eating. Stress and obesity have also been identified as potential factors to acid reflux, confounding the picture of this complex disorder. Heartburn is a burning sensation in the chest that occurs frequently after meals or after lying down. Acid reflux can cause a number of symptoms, including sour-tasting liquid regurgitation, trouble swallowing, and persistent coughing, as well as chest pain, hoarseness, and even teeth erosion. These different presentations highlight the necessity of understanding acid reflux's broad impact on general health and well-being.

Regardless of its prevalence, acid reflux is not a one-size-fits-all condition. Indeed, its manifestations differ widely from person to person, demanding a tailored approach to management and treatment. Individuals can better navigate their route to relief by learning more about the underlying mechanisms that cause acid reflux, arming them with the knowledge and resources they need to make informed decisions that support digestive health. As we continue our investigation into the complexities of acid reflux, it is critical to understand the dynamic interaction of numerous elements that contribute to its start and severity. While diet and lifestyle habits undoubtedly influence our digestive health, it is also critical to consider the impact of physiological factors such as anatomical abnormalities, hormonal imbalances, and genetic predispositions on the onset and progression of reflux symptoms.

Anatomical anomalies, such as a hiatal hernia, in which a piece of the stomach protrudes through the diaphragm into the chest cavity, can weaken the lower esophageal sphincter, increasing the risk of acid reflux. Similarly, hormonal shifts, particularly during pregnancy, can relax the muscles of the esophagus and stomach, causing reflux episodes in vulnerable individuals. Furthermore, hereditary factors may predispose some people to increased acid sensitivity or reduced esophageal motility, complicating the treatment of reflux symptoms. Beyond these physiological concerns, the importance of nutrition and lifestyle in controlling acid reflux cannot be emphasized. Certain foods and beverages, including spicy dishes, citrus fruits, tomatoes, chocolate, caffeinated beverages, and alcohol, are well-known for causing reflux symptoms in susceptible people. Similarly, lifestyle factors such as smoking, overeating, eating late at night, and lying down just after eating might aggravate acid reflux by relaxing the lower esophageal sphincter and delaying stomach emptying.

However, it is critical to understand that the link between nutrition, lifestyle, and acid reflux is not always clear. While specific foods and activities may cause symptoms in some people, others may find relief from focused dietary changes and lifestyle treatments. This variety emphasizes the significance of taking a personalized approach to acid reflux management—one that considers individual sensitivities, preferences, and goals.

In the subsequent subchapters, we'll delve deeper into the subtleties of acid reflux, examining practical ways for reducing symptoms and regaining control of your digestive destiny. From dietary changes and lifestyle treatments to culinary creativity and meal planning mastery, we'll provide you with the knowledge and resources you need to succeed in the face of reflux-related obstacles. So saddle in and prepare to go on a transformative journey that offers not only reflux relief but also a new sense of vitality and well-being.

Navigating the Reflux Minefield: Charting Your Course to Digestive Comfort

Welcome to the war of reflux triggers and the maze of pain! In this subchapter, we'll put on our information armor and go through the dangerous terrain of acid reflux causes. Consider yourself a bold explorer, equipped not with swords and shields, but with intelligence and insight to cross this treacherous terrain. First and foremost, let us throw some light on the elusive triggers that might unleash the fury of acid reflux. Imagine them as inadvertent behaviors or dietary choices that will set them off. They are like buried mines scattered throughout your regular existence. From spicy foods to acidic beverages, stress to late-night eating, these triggers lie in the background, ready to wreck havoc on your digestive system.

Armed with knowledge, you have the ability to discover and neutralize these reflux mines before they detonate. It's all about learning to detect the warning signs and making strategic changes to your lifestyle and diet. Let's start by highlighting some of the most renowned reflux culprits. Consider spicy foods, which thrill the taste buds but can be harmful to your stomach lining. Then there's caffeine, the beloved stimulant found in coffee and tea, which can set off a chain reaction of acid production and send your reflux into overdrive.

But it's not just about avoiding apparent offenders; even seemingly benign choices might have unanticipated repercussions. Consider carbonated beverages, which appear to be harmless effervescent drinks but can cause a flood of bubbles and abdominal discomfort. Or how about citrus fruits, which are high in vitamin C but also high in acidity, which might irritate your stomach?

Now it's time to devise a strategy for navigating the reflux minefield with ease and elegance. It's all about awareness and moderation—being aware of your triggers and making moderate eating choices. Consider yourself an expert mapper, methodically mapping out the geography of your digestive system. Armed with a pen and parchment, you'll navigate the hazardous minefield, carefully documenting each trigger and obstacle.

Remember, no map is complete without markers to help you find your route. In this subchapter, we'll look at the warning signals of impending danger—a rumble in the stomach, a hot sensation in the chest, and a bitter taste crawling up the throat. These are your body's warning signs, advising you to proceed with caution and modify your route as needed.

As you negotiate the reflux minefield, keep a look out for hidden traps and hazards. It's not just about avoiding obvious triggers; occasionally a mix of seemingly unrelated circumstances might cause a flare-up. Perhaps it's the stress of a hectic workday combined with a hastily grabbed fast-food lunch, or the temptation of a late-night snack followed by a nightcap before bed. Identifying these potential traps will help you avoid danger and stay on track for digestive comfort. Every problem provides an opportunity for development and mastery. With each interaction, you'll improve your ability to identify and avoid reflux causes, honing your skills as a seasoned digestive navigator. And, with "The Complete Acid Reflux Solution Cookbook" as your reliable guide, you'll have the knowledge and tools you need to finally overcome the reflux minefield.

But do not worry, dear traveler, because you are not alone on this treacherous journey. With the direction and support provided by "The Complete Acid Reflux Solution Cookbook," you'll have the tools and resources you need to plan your path to digestive comfort. So put on your cloak of awareness, sharpen your sword of discernment, and ready to battle the reflux minefield once and for all!

Building Your Reflux-Resistant Kitchen: Creating Your Haven of Relief

Welcome to the heart of your home—the kitchen—where we'll go on a revolutionary adventure to create a space that not only satisfies the senses but also provides a safe haven from the discomforts of acid reflux. In this subchapter, we'll look at the detailed process of creating a reflux-resistant kitchen, where every item, tool, and technique is carefully chosen to benefit your digestive health.

Let's start with the basics: your pantry. Open the doors to discover a bounty of reflux-friendly items that will serve as the foundation for your culinary masterpieces. From complete grains like quinoa and brown rice to lean proteins like chicken and fish, stocking your cupboard with nourishing staples ensures that you always have the ingredients for nutritious, reflux-friendly meals on hand. A acid-resistant kitchen, however, consists of more than simply well-stocked shelves; it also includes smart substitutes and strategic swaps that reduce the danger of triggering reflux symptoms. Say goodbye to acidic condiments like vinegar and citrus juices, and welcome to milder alternatives like apple cider vinegar and lemon zest. Embrace the variety of herbs and spices to add depth and flavor to your foods without using excessive salt or fat.

As we progress from the pantry to the fridge and freezer, we'll discover a plethora of options for maintaining freshness and increasing flavor. Learn how to batch cook and meal prep so that you always have healthful, homemade meals on hand to enjoy at any time. Discover the convenience of frozen fruits and veggies, which keep nutritious content while also providing a quick and easy way to add color and diversity to your meals. Perhaps the most important aspect of your reflux-resistant kitchen are the tools and equipment that allow for easy cooking and cleanup. Invest in high-quality cookware and utensils to ensure uniform cooking and reduce the need for additional fats and oils. Explore the world of kitchen gadgets and equipment, from blenders and food processors to air fryers and slow cookers, that will make meal preparation easier and broaden your culinary horizons. Let's explore deeper into the complexities of designing your reflux-resistant kitchen by looking at other strategies and insights that will improve your culinary experience and your digestive health.

Organization is essential for productivity and convenience in the kitchen. Take the time to tidy and arrange your environment, making sure that everything has a dedicated spot and is easily accessible. Invest in storage solutions such as clear containers and labeled jars to keep your ingredients visible and organized, minimizing meal prep stress and sparking culinary innovation. When stocking your cupboard with reflux-friendly staples, remember to evaluate the quality of the components. Choose organic produce wherever possible to reduce your exposure to pesticides and other dangerous chemicals. Choose whole, minimally processed foods over refined ones to enhance nutritional content and support overall digestive health. When it comes to culinary methods, simplicity is typically preferred. Use moderate cooking methods such as steaming, poaching, and baking to maintain the natural flavors and textures of your ingredients without adding extra fat or salt. Experiment with herbs, spices, and aromatics to give your recipes depth and complexity without using sour or hot ingredients.

Incorporating probiotic-rich foods into your diet can also help improve gut health and reduce reflux symptoms. Stock your refrigerator with fermented foods such as yogurt, kefir, sauerkraut, and kimchi to create a healthy gut bacteria balance and boost your body's natural defenses against digestive pain. Aside from the physical aspects of your kitchen, developing a mindful attitude to cooking and eating can improve your digestive health. Take the time to take each bite, noticing the flavors, textures, and feelings that emerge. Practice mindful eating practices such as chewing gently, putting down utensils between bites, and paying attention to your body's hunger and fullness signs. As you continue to develop and evolve your reflux-resistant kitchen, may it provide you with comfort, inspiration, and empowerment as you work toward good digestive health. With each wonderful meal you prepare, may you discover the transformative power of food to heal, nourish, and restore balance to your body and soul. As you finish your reflux-resistant kitchen, take a moment to enjoy the sense of success that comes from knowing you've created a home that nurtures both body and soul.

Finally, remember to fill your kitchen with love and intention. Cooking is more than just fueling the body; it is also a means of self-expression and communication with loved ones. Invite friends and family to join you in the kitchen and share the delight of cooking and eating together. Cultivate thankfulness for the quantity of nutritious meals at your disposal, and approach each meal with a sense of wonder, creativity, and appreciation.

Chapter 2

Rise and Shine: Breakfast Solutions

Mornings can be tough, especially when you're battling acid reflux. But fear not! In this chapter, we'll explore a plethora of breakfast solutions that not only kickstart your day but also soothe your stomach and set the tone for a comfortable morning. From light and refreshing options to hearty classics, there's something here to suit every palate and every level of hunger.

Start your day with a burst of flavor and nutrition with our selection of fruit-packed smoothies. Blend up a refreshing concoction of bananas, strawberries, and almond milk for a creamy treat that's gentle on the stomach yet invigorating for the senses. Or opt for a tropical twist with a pineapple and coconut water blend that transports you to a sunny beach with every sip. If you prefer something more substantial, our oatmeal variations are sure to satisfy. Dive into a comforting bowl of warm oats topped with sliced bananas, a drizzle of honey, and a sprinkle of cinnamon for a breakfast that feels like a hug in a bowl. Or get adventurous with savory oatmeal topped with avocado, cherry tomatoes, and a poached egg for a protein-packed start to your day.

For those who crave a bit of indulgence in the morning, our selection of baked goods is sure to please. From fluffy pancakes drizzled with maple syrup to flaky pastries filled with fruit compote, these breakfast treats are guaranteed to satisfy your sweet tooth without aggravating your reflux symptoms. Pair them with a cup of soothing herbal tea or a glass of almond milk for the perfect morning indulgence.

And let's not forget about the power of eggs! Whether scrambled, poached, or sunny-side-up, eggs are a versatile and nutritious addition to any breakfast spread. Whip up a veggie-packed omelet or serve it atop whole grain toast for a protein-rich meal that keeps you full and focused until lunchtime.

No matter your breakfast preference, our breakfast solutions are designed to nourish your body and soothe your stomach, setting you up for a day of digestive ease and culinary delight. So, rise and shine with confidence, knowing that your first meal of the day is both delicious and reflux-friendly.

Fruit-packed Smoothies

Banana Berry Bliss:
- Ingredients: Bananas, strawberries, blueberries, almond milk
- Instructions: Blend together bananas, strawberries, blueberries, and almond milk for a refreshing and satisfying smoothie.

Mango Tango:
- Ingredients: Ripe mangoes, pineapple chunks, coconut water
- Instructions: Combine ripe mangoes, pineapple chunks, and coconut water for a tropical treat that's gentle on the stomach.

Peachy Keen:
- Ingredients: Peaches, raspberries, Greek yogurt
- Instructions: Blend peaches, raspberries, and Greek yogurt for a creamy and delicious smoothie with a hint of tartness.

Berry Blast:
- Ingredients: Variety of berries (strawberries, raspberries, and blackberries); a splash of orange juice
- Instructions: Mix together a variety of berries, such as strawberries, raspberries, and blackberries, with a splash of orange juice for a burst of flavor.

Tropical Paradise:
- Ingredients: Pineapple, mango, kiwi, coconut milk
- Instructions: Blend together pineapple, mango, kiwi, and coconut milk for a refreshing smoothie reminiscent of a day at the beach.

Green Goddess:
- Ingredients: Spinach, kale, banana, pineapple, coconut water
- Instructions: Combine spinach, kale, banana, pineapple, and coconut water for a nutrient-rich smoothie that's easy on the stomach.

Citrus Sunrise:
- Ingredients: Oranges, bananas, hint of ginger
- Instructions: Blend oranges, bananas, and a hint of ginger for a zesty and invigorating smoothie to start your day.

Strawberry Banana Delight:
- Ingredients: Ripe strawberries, bananas, Greek yogurt
- Instructions: Mix ripe strawberries, bananas, and a dollop of Greek yogurt for a creamy and satisfying smoothie.

Blueberry Blast:
- Ingredients: Blueberries, bananas, almond milk
- Instructions: Blend blueberries, bananas, and almond milk for an antioxidant-rich smoothie that's as delicious as it is nutritious.

Pineapple Paradise:
- Ingredients: Pineapple, bananas, coconut water
- Instructions: Combine pineapple, bananas, and coconut water for a tropical smoothie that transports you to the islands.

Kiwi Kiss:
- Blend 2 ripe kiwis, 1 ripe banana, and a splash of lime juice until smooth.
- Enjoy this refreshing and tangy smoothie as a revitalizing start to your day.

Raspberry Dream:
- Mix 1 cup of fresh raspberries, 1 ripe banana, and ½ cup of Greek yogurt until creamy.
- Indulge in this creamy and indulgent smoothie with a hint of tartness for a satisfying treat.

Mango Madness:
- Combine 1 ripe mango, 1 ripe banana, and ½ cup of coconut milk in a blender.

- Blend until creamy and enjoy the burst of tropical flavor in this creamy smoothie.

Berry Banana Bonanza:
- Blend a mix of berries (such as strawberries, blueberries, and raspberries), 1 ripe banana, and 1 cup of almond milk until smooth.
- Savor the delicious and satisfying blend of berries and banana in this creamy smoothie.

Peach Perfection:
- Mix 2 ripe peaches, 1 ripe banana, and a splash of orange juice in a blender until smooth.
- Enjoy the sweet and refreshing taste of this smoothie for a perfect start to your morning.

Green Goodness:
- Combine a handful of spinach, 1 ripe kiwi, 1 cup of pineapple chunks, and ½ cup of coconut water in a blender.
- Blend until smooth for a nutrient-packed smoothie that's both healthy and delicious.

Strawberry Pineapple Paradise:
- Blend 1 cup of fresh strawberries, 1 cup of pineapple chunks, and ½ cup of coconut milk until smooth.
- Transport yourself to a tropical paradise with this refreshing and fruity smoothie.

Blueberry Banana Bliss:
- Mix 1 cup of blueberries, 1 ripe banana, and ½ cup of Greek yogurt in a blender until creamy.
- Enjoy the antioxidant-rich goodness of blueberries in this creamy and satisfying smoothie.

Mango Coconut Crush:
- Combine 1 ripe mango, ½ cup of coconut milk, and a splash of lime juice in a blender.
- Blend until smooth for a tropical treat that's gentle on the stomach.

Berry Beet Blast
- Blend a mix of berries with cooked beets and 1 cup of almond milk until smooth.
- Enjoy the vibrant color and nutrient-rich goodness of this smoothie.

Pineapple Spinach Surprise:
- Mix pineapple, spinach, bananas, and coconut water in a blender.
- Blend until smooth and creamy.
- Pour into a glass and enjoy this refreshing and nutrient-packed smoothie.

Kiwi Berry Burst:
- Combine kiwi, mixed berries, and Greek yogurt in a blender.
- Blend until smooth and creamy.
- Pour into a glass and savor the tangy and creamy flavors of this smoothie.

Raspberry Lime Refresher:
- Blend raspberries, lime juice, and bananas in a blender.
- Blend until smooth and creamy.
- Pour into a glass and refresh yourself with the zesty and invigorating flavors of this smoothie.

Orange Creamsicle:
- Mix oranges, bananas, and vanilla Greek yogurt in a blender.
- Blend until smooth and creamy.
- Pour into a glass and indulge in the creamy and citrusy nostalgia of this childhood favorite.

Strawberry Mango Madness:
- Blend strawberries, mangoes, and coconut water in a blender.
- Blend until smooth and creamy.
- Pour into a glass and immerse yourself in the tropical burst of flavor of this smoothie.

Blueberry Coconut Cooler:
- Combine blueberries, coconut milk, and a splash of lime juice in a blender.
- Blend until smooth and creamy.
- Pour into a glass and cool off with the refreshing and antioxidant-rich blend of flavors.

Pineapple Kale Powerhouse:
- Blend pineapple, kale, bananas, and almond milk in a blender.
- Blend until smooth and creamy.
- Pour into a glass and fuel your day with the nutrient-packed goodness of this smoothie with a tropical twist.

Peach Raspberry Revitalizer:
- Mix peaches, raspberries, and Greek yogurt in a blender.
- Blend until smooth and creamy.
- Pour into a glass and rejuvenate your senses with the creamy and refreshing blend of flavors.

Berry Banana Coconut Crush:
- Blend mixed berries, bananas, and coconut milk in a blender.
- Blend until smooth and creamy.
- Pour into a glass and enjoy the creamy and tropical explosion of flavors in this smoothie.

Mango Spinach Surprise:
- Combine ripe mangoes, spinach, and coconut water in a blender.
- Blend until smooth and creamy.

- Pour into a glass and savor the nutrient-packed goodness with a hint of sweetness in this smoothie.

Orange Carrot Concoction:
- Ingredients: Oranges, carrots, and ginger
- Instructions: Blend together oranges, carrots, and a splash of ginger until smooth. Enjoy this vibrant and refreshing smoothie with a hint of spice.

Strawberry Pineapple Basil Bliss:
- Ingredients: Strawberries, pineapple, fresh basil leaves, coconut water
- Instructions: Mix strawberries, pineapple, fresh basil leaves, and coconut water in a blender until smooth. Savor the unique and refreshing flavors of this smoothie.

Blueberry Almond Butter Delight:
- Ingredients: Blueberries, almond butter, bananas, almond milk
- Instructions: Combine blueberries, almond butter, bananas, and almond milk in a blender. Blend until creamy and enjoy this protein-rich smoothie.

Pineapple Coconut Green Goddess:
- Ingredients: Pineapple, coconut milk, spinach, bananas
- Instructions: Blend together pineapple, coconut milk, spinach, and bananas until smooth. Indulge in this tropical and nutrient-packed smoothie.

Kiwi Mango Madness:
- Ingredients: Kiwi, mangoes, coconut water
- Instructions: Mix kiwi, mangoes, and coconut water in a blender until well combined. Sip on this refreshing and tropical smoothie with a tangy twist.

Raspberry Peach Perfection:
- Ingredients: Raspberries, peaches, Greek yogurt
- Instructions: Blend raspberries, peaches, and Greek yogurt until smooth and creamy. Enjoy this satisfying smoothie with a hint of tartness.

Blueberry Cherry Blast:
- Ingredients: Blueberries, cherries, almond milk
- Instructions: Combine blueberries, cherries, and almond milk in a blender. Blend until smooth and relish in the antioxidant-rich burst of flavor.

Pineapple Banana Coconut Cream:
- Ingredients: Pineapple, bananas, coconut milk, vanilla extract
- Instructions: Blend pineapple, bananas, coconut milk, and a splash of vanilla extract until creamy and smooth. Delight in this creamy and tropical treat.

Mango Strawberry Surprise:
- Ingredients: Ripe mangoes, strawberries, Greek yogurt
- Instructions: Mix ripe mangoes, strawberries, and Greek yogurt in a blender until smooth and refreshing. Savor the delightful combination of flavors.

Mixed Berry Chia Delight:
- Ingredients: Mixed berries, chia seeds, bananas, almond milk
- Instructions: Blend mixed berries, chia seeds, bananas, and almond milk until smooth and creamy. Enjoy this fiber-rich and satisfying smoothie.

Papaya Pineapple Paradise:
- Ingredients: Papaya, pineapple, coconut water, lime juice
- Instructions: Combine papaya, pineapple, coconut water, and a splash of lime juice in a blender. Blend until smooth and relish in this tropical and refreshing smoothie.

Blackberry Banana Bliss:
- Ingredients: Blackberries, bananas, Greek yogurt
- Instructions: Blend blackberries, bananas, and Greek yogurt until creamy and antioxidant-rich. Indulge in this satisfying and nutritious smoothie.

Mango Avocado Dream:
- Ingredients: Ripe mangoes, avocado, coconut milk, lime juice
- Instructions: Mix ripe mangoes, avocado, coconut milk, and a splash of lime juice in a blender until smooth and creamy. Enjoy this nutrient-packed and creamy smoothie.

Peach Raspberry Coconut Cooler:
- Ingredients: Peaches, raspberries, coconut milk, lime juice
- Instructions: Combine peaches, raspberries, coconut milk, and a splash of lime juice in a blender. Blend until smooth and refreshing. Sip on this tropical and cooling smoothie.

Blueberry Mango Madness:
- Ingredients: Blueberries, ripe mangoes, Greek yogurt
- Instructions: Blend blueberries, ripe mangoes, and Greek yogurt until smooth and creamy. Enjoy this antioxidant-rich and flavorful smoothie.

Oatmeal Variations

===

Classic Cinnamon Banana Oatmeal:

Ingredients:
- Oats
- Sliced bananas
- Ground cinnamon
- Honey

Instructions:

1. Cook oats according to package instructions.
2. Top cooked oats with sliced bananas.
3. Sprinkle it with ground cinnamon.
4. Drizzle with honey.
5. Stir well and enjoy!

===

Berry Blast Oatmeal:

Ingredients:
- Oats
- Fresh or frozen berries (strawberries, blueberries, raspberries)

Instructions:

1. Cook the oats according to the package instructions.
2. Mix in a handful of fresh or frozen berries.
3. Stir well to combine.
4. Serve and enjoy the burst of antioxidants and natural sweetness!

===

Apple Cinnamon Oatmeal:

Ingredients:
- Oats
- Diced apples
- Ground cinnamon

Instructions:

1. Cook oats according to package instructions.
2. Stir in diced apples.
3. Sprinkle it with ground cinnamon.
4. Mix well and savor the cozy flavors of autumn!

===

Peachy Keen Oatmeal:

Ingredients:
- Oats
- Diced peaches

- Vanilla extract

Instructions:

1. Cook oats according to package instructions.
2. Add diced peaches to the cooked oats.
3. Stir in a touch of vanilla extract for a fruity and aromatic twist.
4. Enjoy the taste of summer in every bite!

Tropical Oatmeal Delight:

Ingredients:

- Oats
- Diced pineapple
- Shredded coconut
- Chopped macadamia nuts

Instructions:

1. Cook oats according to package instructions.
2. Mix in diced pineapple, shredded coconut, and chopped macadamia nuts.
3. Stir well to combine.
4. Close your eyes and imagine yourself on a tropical island paradise as you enjoy this delightful oatmeal!

Almond Joy Oatmeal:

Ingredients:

- Oats
- Almond butter
- Shredded coconut
- Dark chocolate

Instructions:

1. Cook oats according to package instructions.
2. Stir in almond butter and shredded coconut.
3. Drizzle with melted dark chocolate.
4. Mix well and indulge in this decadent morning treat reminiscent of your favorite candy bar!

Pumpkin Spice Oatmeal:

Ingredients:

- Oats
- Canned pumpkin puree
- Pumpkin pie spice
- Greek yogurt

Instructions:

1. Cook oats according to package instructions.
2. Stir in canned pumpkin puree and pumpkin pie spice.
3. Top with a dollop of Greek yogurt for creaminess.
4. Enjoy the cozy flavors of fall in every spoonful!

Lemon Blueberry Oatmeal:

Ingredients:

- Oats
- Fresh or frozen blueberries
- Fresh lemon juice

Instructions:

1. Cook oats according to package instructions.
2. Mix in fresh or frozen blueberries.
3. Squeeze fresh lemon juice over the oatmeal.
4. Stir well and savor the refreshing and tangy flavors!

Cherry Almond Oatmeal:

Ingredients:

- Oats
- Chopped cherries
- Slivered almonds

Instructions:

1. Cook oats according to package instructions.
2. Stir in chopped cherries and slivered almonds.
3. Mix well and enjoy the deliciously nutty and slightly tart flavors!

Peanut Butter Banana Oatmeal:

- **Ingredients:**
- Oats
- Creamy peanut butter
- Sliced bananas

Instructions:

1. Cook oats according to package instructions.
2. Swirl in creamy peanut butter.
3. Add sliced bananas.
4. Stir well to combine.
5. Enjoy this protein-packed and satisfying morning meal!

=====

Chocolate Banana Oatmeal:

Ingredients:

- Oats
- Cocoa powder
- Sliced bananas
- Honey

Instructions:

1. Cook oats according to package instructions.
2. Stir in cocoa powder until well combined.
3. Top with sliced bananas.
4. Drizzle with honey before serving.

=====

Maple Pecan Oatmeal:

Ingredients:

- Oats
- Chopped pecans
- Maple syrup

Instructions:

1. Cook the oats according to the package instructions.
2. Mix in chopped pecans.

3. Drizzle with maple syrup before serving.

=====

Fig and Honey Oatmeal:
Ingredients:

- Oats
- Diced dried figs
- Honey

Instructions:

1. Cook oats according to package instructions.
2. Stir in diced dried figs.
3. Drizzle with honey before serving.

=====

Coconut Mango Oatmeal:

Ingredients:

- Oats
- Diced mango
- Shredded coconut

Instructions:

1. Cook the oats according to the package instructions.

2. Mix in diced mango and shredded coconut before serving.

Raspberry Almond Oatmeal:

Ingredients:

- Oats
- Fresh raspberries
- Slivered almonds

Instructions:

1. Cook the oats according to package instructions.
2. Top with fresh raspberries and slivered almonds before serving.

Blueberry Lemon Poppy Seed Oatmeal:

Ingredients:

- Oats
- Fresh blueberries
- Lemon zest
- Poppy seeds

Instructions:

1. Cook oats according to package instructions.
2. Mix in fresh blueberries, lemon zest, and poppy seeds before serving.

Vanilla Bean Oatmeal:

Ingredients:

- Oats
- Vanilla bean paste or vanilla extract

Instructions:

1. Cook oats according to package instructions.
2. Stir in vanilla bean paste or vanilla extract before serving.

Maple Walnut Oatmeal:

Ingredients:

- Oats
- Chopped walnuts
- Maple syrup

Instructions:

1. Cook oats according to package instructions.
2. Mix in chopped walnuts.
3. Drizzle with maple syrup before serving.

Cranberry Orange Oatmeal:

Ingredients:

- Oats
- Dried cranberries
- Fresh orange zest
- Orange juice

Instructions:

1. Cook oats according to package instructions.
2. Add dried cranberries and fresh orange zest.
3. Squeeze orange juice over the oatmeal before serving.

Pistachio Cardamom Oatmeal:

Ingredients:

- Oats
- Chopped pistachios
- Ground cardamom

Instructions:

1. Cook oats according to package instructions.
2. Stir in chopped pistachios and ground cardamom before serving.

Strawberry Rhubarb Oatmeal:

- ### Ingredients:
    1. Oats
    2. Diced strawberries
    3. Cooked rhubarb
- ### Instructions:
1. Cook oats according to package instructions.
2. Mix in diced strawberries and cooked rhubarb before serving.

Hazelnut Chocolate Oatmeal:

Ingredients:

- Oats
- Chopped hazelnuts
- Dark chocolate chips

Instructions:

1. Cook oats according to package instructions.

2. Add chopped hazelnuts and a sprinkle of dark chocolate chips before serving.

Maple Bacon Oatmeal:

Ingredients:

- Oats
- Cooked bacon, crumbled
- Maple syrup

Instructions:

1. Cook oats according to package instructions.
2. Sprinkle crumbled cooked bacon over the oatmeal.
3. Drizzle with maple syrup before serving.

Pina Colada Oatmeal:

Ingredients:

- Oats
- Diced pineapple
- Shredded coconut
- Coconut milk

Instructions:

1. Cook oats according to package instructions.
2. Mix in diced pineapple and shredded coconut.
3. Add a splash of coconut milk before serving.

Matcha Green Tea Oatmeal:

Ingredients:

- Oats
- Matcha powder

Instructions:

1. Cook oats according to package instructions.
2. Stir in matcha powder before serving for a vibrant green color and earthy flavor profile.

Breakfast Veggie Variations

Spinach and Mushroom Omelet:

Ingredients:

- 2 cups fresh spinach leaves
- 1 cup sliced mushrooms
- 3 eggs
- Salt and pepper to taste
- Olive oil or butter for sautéing

Instructions:

1. Heat a drizzle of olive oil or a pat of butter in a skillet over medium heat.
2. Add the sliced mushrooms to the skillet and cook until they start to brown, about 3-4 minutes.
3. Add the fresh spinach leaves to the skillet and cook until wilted, about 2-3 minutes.
4. In a separate bowl, beat the eggs and season with salt and pepper.
5. Pour the beaten eggs over the sautéed spinach and mushrooms in the skillet.
6. Allow the eggs to cook undisturbed until the edges start to set, then gently fold the omelet in half.
7. Continue cooking until the eggs are fully set and cooked through.
8. Serve hot and enjoy your nutritious and reflux-friendly spinach and mushroom omelet!

Zucchini Fritters:

Ingredients:

- 2 medium zucchinis, grated
- 2 eggs
- 1/4 cup breadcrumbs
- Salt and pepper to taste
- Olive oil for frying

Instructions:

1. Place the grated zucchini in a clean kitchen towel and squeeze out any excess moisture.
2. In a mixing bowl, combine the grated zucchini, eggs, breadcrumbs, salt, and pepper.
3. Heat a drizzle of olive oil in a skillet over medium heat.
4. Scoop spoonful of the zucchini mixture into the hot skillet,

flattening them slightly with the back of the spoon.

5. Cook the fritters for 2-3 minutes on each side, or until golden brown and crispy.

6. Transfer the cooked fritters to a plate lined with paper towels to drain any excess oil.

7. Serve hot and enjoy your crunchy and satisfying zucchini fritters!

Bell Pepper and Onion Frittata:

Ingredients:

- 1 bell pepper, diced
- 1 onion, diced
- 6 eggs
- Salt and pepper to taste
- Fresh herbs (such as parsley or chives), chopped
- Olive oil for sautéing

Instructions:

1. Preheat your oven to 350°F (175°C).
2. Heat a drizzle of olive oil in an oven-safe skillet over medium heat.
3. Add the diced bell pepper and onion to the skillet and cook until softened, about 5-7 minutes.
4. In a mixing bowl, beat the eggs and season with salt, pepper, and chopped herbs.
5. Pour the beaten eggs over the sautéed bell pepper and onion in the skillet.
6. Cook the frittata on the stovetop for 2-3 minutes, then transfer the skillet to the preheated oven.
7. Bake the frittata for 10-12 minutes, or until the eggs are set and cooked through.
8. Remove the skillet from the oven and let the frittata cool slightly before slicing and serving.
9. Enjoy your colorful and flavorful bell pepper and onion frittata for a delicious breakfast option!

Avocado Toast

Ingredients:

- 1 ripe avocado
- 2 slices whole grain bread
- 1 tomato, sliced
- Salt and pepper to taste

Instructions:

1. Toast the slices of whole grain bread until golden brown and crispy.

2. While the bread is toasting, halve the avocado, remove the pit, and scoop the flesh into a bowl.
3. Use a fork to mash the avocado until smooth and creamy.
4. Spread the mashed avocado evenly onto the toasted bread slices.
5. Top each avocado toast with sliced tomatoes.
6. Season with salt and pepper to taste.
7. Serve immediately and enjoy your simple yet satisfying avocado toast!

Cauliflower Hash Browns

Ingredients:

- 2 cups grated cauliflower
- 2 eggs
- 1/4 cup breadcrumbs
- 1/4 teaspoon garlic powder
- Salt and pepper to taste
- Olive oil for frying

Instructions:

1. Place the grated cauliflower in a clean kitchen towel and squeeze out any excess moisture.
2. In a mixing bowl, combine the grated cauliflower, eggs, breadcrumbs, garlic powder, salt, and pepper.
3. Heat a drizzle of olive oil in a skillet over medium heat.
4. Scoop spoonful of the cauliflower mixture into the hot skillet, flattening them slightly with the back of the spoon to form patties.
5. Cook the hash browns for 3-4 minutes on each side, or until golden brown and crispy.
6. Transfer the cooked hash browns to a plate lined with paper towels to drain any excess oil.
7. Serve hot and enjoy your low-carb cauliflower hash browns!

Broccoli and Cheese Quiche

Ingredients:

- 1 cup broccoli florets, chopped
- 1/2 cup shredded sharp cheddar cheese
- 4 eggs
- 1/2 cup milk (or dairy-free alternative)
- Salt and pepper to taste
- Pie crust (store-bought or homemade)

Instructions:

1. Preheat your oven to 375ºF (190ºC).
2. Roll out the pie crust and line a pie dish with it, trimming any excess dough.
3. In a mixing bowl, beat the eggs and milk together until well combined.
4. Stir in the chopped broccoli florets and shredded cheddar cheese.
5. Season the mixture with salt and pepper to taste.
6. Pour the broccoli and cheese mixture into the prepared pie crust.
7. Bake the quiche in the preheated oven for 30-35 minutes, or until the filling is set and the crust is golden brown.
8. Remove the quiche from the oven and let it cool slightly before slicing and serving.
9. Enjoy your hearty and flavorful broccoli and cheese quiche for a delicious breakfast or brunch!

Tomato and Basil Frittata:

Ingredients:

- 1 cup cherry tomatoes, halved
- 1/4 cup fresh basil leaves, chopped
- 4 eggs
- 1/4 cup grated Parmesan cheese
- Salt and pepper to taste

- Olive oil for sautéing

Instructions:

1. Preheat your oven to 350ºF (175ºC).
2. Heat a drizzle of olive oil in an oven-safe skillet over medium heat.
3. Add the cherry tomatoes to the skillet and cook until they start to soften, about 3-4 minutes.
4. Stir in the chopped fresh basil leaves and cook for an additional 1-2 minutes.
5. In a mixing bowl, beat the eggs and grated Parmesan cheese together until well combined.
6. Season the egg mixture with salt and pepper to taste.
7. Pour the egg mixture over the sautéed tomatoes and basil in the skillet.

8. Cook the frittata on the stovetop for 2-3 minutes, then transfer the skillet to the preheated oven.
9. Bake the frittata for 10-12 minutes, or until the eggs are set and cooked through.
10. Remove the skillet from the oven and let the frittata cool slightly before slicing and serving.

11. Enjoy your burst of Italian flavor in every bite with this tomato and basil frittata!

Asparagus and Goat Cheese Omelet:

Ingredients:

- 1/2 cup asparagus spears, trimmed and cut into bite-sized pieces
- 2 eggs
- 2 tablespoons crumbled goat cheese
- Salt and pepper to taste
- Olive oil or butter for sautéing

Instructions:

1. Heat a drizzle of olive oil or a pat of butter in a skillet over medium heat.
2. Add the trimmed asparagus spears to the skillet and cook until they are tender-crisp, about 3-4 minutes.
3. In a bowl, beat the eggs and season with salt and pepper.
4. Pour the beaten eggs into the skillet over the asparagus.
5. Cook the eggs until the edges start to set, then sprinkle the crumbled goat cheese over one half of the omelet.
6. Gently fold the other half of the omelet over the cheese, forming a half-moon shape.
7. Continue cooking until the eggs are fully set and the cheese is melted.
8. Slide the omelet onto a plate and serve hot, savoring the creamy goat cheese and tender-crisp asparagus in every bite.

Spinach and Feta Breakfast Wrap:

Ingredients:

- 1 whole grain wrap or tortilla
- 1/2 cup fresh spinach leaves
- 2 tablespoons crumbled feta cheese
- 2 eggs, scrambled
- Salt and pepper to taste

Instructions:

1. Heat the whole grain wrap in a dry skillet over medium heat for a few seconds on each side to warm it up.
2. Place the warmed wrap on a plate or flat surface.
3. Arrange the fresh spinach leaves in the center of the wrap.
4. Sprinkle the crumbled feta cheese over the spinach.
5. Spoon the scrambled eggs on top of the spinach and feta.
6. Season with salt and pepper to taste.
7. Fold in the sides of the wrap, then roll it up tightly from the bottom to form a wrap.
8. Slice the wrap in half diagonally, if desired, and serve warm for a portable and nutritious breakfast option.

Mushroom and Swiss Cheese Omelet:

Ingredients:

- 1/2 cup sliced mushrooms
- 1/4 cup diced onions
- 2 eggs
- 1/4 cup shredded Swiss cheese
- Salt and pepper to taste
- Olive oil or butter for sautéing

Instructions:

1. Heat a drizzle of olive oil or a pat of butter in a skillet over medium heat.
2. Add the sliced mushrooms and diced onions to the skillet and cook until they are tender and golden brown, about 5-7 minutes.
3. In a bowl, beat the eggs and season with salt and pepper.
4. Pour the beaten eggs into the skillet over the cooked mushrooms and onions.
5. Allow the eggs to cook undisturbed until the edges start to set, then sprinkle the shredded Swiss cheese over one half of the omelet.
6. Gently fold the other half of the omelet over the cheese, forming a half-moon shape.
7. Continue cooking until the eggs are fully set and the cheese is melted.
8. Slide the omelet onto a plate and serve hot, enjoying the savory combination of mushrooms, onions, and Swiss cheese in every bite.

Veggie Breakfast Burrito:

Ingredients:

- 1 whole grain tortilla
- 2 eggs, scrambled
- 1/4 cup diced bell peppers
- 1/4 cup diced onions
- 2 tablespoons salsa
- Salt and pepper to taste

Instructions:

1. Warm the whole grain tortilla in a dry skillet over medium heat for a few seconds on each side to make it pliable.
2. Place the warmed tortilla on a plate or flat surface.
3. Spoon the scrambled eggs onto the center of the tortilla.
4. Sprinkle the diced bell peppers and onions over the scrambled eggs.
5. Drizzle the salsa over the vegetables and eggs.
6. Season with salt and pepper to taste.
7. Fold in the sides of the tortilla, then roll it up tightly from the bottom to form a burrito.
8. Slice the burrito in half diagonally, if desired, and serve warm for a flavorful and filling breakfast on the go.

Eggplant and Tomato Scramble:

Ingredients:

- 1 small eggplant, diced
- 1 cup cherry tomatoes, halved
- 2 cloves garlic, minced
- 2 eggs
- Salt and pepper to taste
- Olive oil for sautéing
- Fresh herbs (such as basil or parsley) for garnish (optional)

Instructions:

1. Heat a drizzle of olive oil in a skillet over medium heat.
2. Add the diced eggplant to the skillet and cook until it starts to soften and brown, about 5-7 minutes.
3. Add the halved cherry tomatoes and minced garlic to the skillet with the eggplant and cook for an additional 2-3 minutes, until the tomatoes are slightly softened.
4. In a bowl, beat the eggs and season with salt and pepper.

5. Pour the beaten eggs into the skillet over the cooked vegetables.
6. Stir the mixture gently and continuously until the eggs are cooked to your desired consistency and everything is well combined.
7. Transfer the scramble to a plate and garnish with fresh herbs if desired.

8. Serve hot and enjoy the Mediterranean-inspired flavors of this eggplant and tomato scramble!

Sweet Potato Hash:

Ingredients:

- 1 large sweet potato, peeled and diced
- 1/2 cup diced onions
- 1/2 cup diced bell peppers
- 2 tablespoons olive oil
- Salt and pepper to taste

- Fresh herbs (such as parsley or thyme) for garnish (optional)

Instructions:

1. Heat the olive oil in a skillet over medium heat.
2. Add the diced sweet potatoes to the skillet and cook until they are golden brown and tender, about 10-12 minutes, stirring occasionally.
3. Add the diced onions and bell peppers to the skillet with the cooked sweet potatoes and cook for an additional 3-4 minutes, until the vegetables are softened.
4. Season the hash with salt and pepper to taste, and garnish with fresh herbs if desired.

5. Serve hot and enjoy the hearty and satisfying flavors of this sweet potato hash for a nutritious breakfast option!

Kale and Tomato Omelet:

Ingredients:

- 1 cup chopped kale leaves
- 1/2 cup cherry tomatoes, halved
- 2 eggs
- Salt and pepper to taste
- Olive oil for sautéing

- Grated Parmesan cheese for garnish (optional)

Instructions:

1. Heat a drizzle of olive oil in a skillet over medium heat.
2. Add the chopped kale leaves to the skillet and cook until they are wilted, about 2-3 minutes.
3. Add the halved cherry tomatoes to the skillet with the kale and cook for an additional 1-2 minutes, until the tomatoes are slightly softened.
4. In a bowl, beat the eggs and season with salt and pepper.
5. Pour the beaten eggs into the skillet over the cooked vegetables.
6. Allow the eggs to cook undisturbed until the edges start to set, then gently lift the edges of the omelet and tilt the skillet to let the uncooked eggs flow to the edges.
7. Once the eggs are mostly set but still slightly runny on top, sprinkle grated Parmesan cheese over one half of the omelet.
8. Gently fold the other half of the omelet over the cheese, forming a half-moon shape.
9. Continue cooking until the eggs are fully set and the cheese is melted.
10. Slide the omelet onto a plate and serve hot, garnished with additional Parmesan cheese if desired.

Roasted Vegetable Breakfast Bowl:

Ingredients:

- 2 cups mixed roasted vegetables (such as carrots, Brussels sprouts, and squash)
- 1 cup cooked quinoa or brown rice
- 2 eggs, poached or fried
- Salt and pepper to taste
- Fresh herbs (such as cilantro or parsley) for garnish (optional)

- Hot sauce or salsa for serving (optional)

Instructions:

1. Preheat your oven to 400°F (200°C).
2. Toss the mixed vegetables with a drizzle of olive oil, salt, and pepper on a baking sheet.

3. Roast the vegetables in the preheated oven for 20-25 minutes, or until they are tender and caramelized, stirring halfway through cooking.
4. Divide the cooked quinoa or brown rice between serving bowls.
5. Top each bowl with a portion of the roasted vegetables.
6. Cook the eggs to your liking (poached or fried) and place one egg on top of each bowl.
7. Season the bowls with salt and pepper to taste, and garnish with fresh herbs if desired.
8. Serve hot, with hot sauce or salsa on the side if desired, and enjoy the hearty and satisfying flavors of this roasted vegetable breakfast bowl!

Carrot and Ginger Smoothie:

Ingredients:

- 1 large carrot, peeled and chopped
- 1-inch piece of fresh ginger, peeled and grated
- 1 ripe banana
- 1 cup almond milk

Instructions:

1. Place chopped carrot, grated ginger, banana, and almond milk in a blender.
2. Blend until smooth and creamy.
3. Pour into a glass and serve immediately

Spaghetti Squash Breakfast Bowl:

Ingredients:

- 1 small spaghetti squash
- 4 large eggs
- 1 cup diced tomatoes
- 1/4 cup fresh basil, chopped
- Salt and pepper, to taste

Instructions:

1. Preheat the oven to 400°F (200°C).
2. Cut spaghetti squash in half lengthwise and remove seeds.
3. Place squash halves cut side down on a baking sheet lined with parchment paper.
4. Bake for 30-40 minutes or until squash is tender and easily pierced with a fork.
5. While squash is baking, scramble eggs in a skillet until cooked through.

6. Use a fork to scrape the cooked spaghetti squash into a bowl.
7. Top with scrambled eggs, diced tomatoes, chopped fresh basil, salt, and pepper.
8. Serve hot as a low-carb and satisfying breakfast bowl.

Pea and Mint Frittata:

Ingredients:

- 6 large eggs
- 1 cup fresh or frozen peas
- 2 tablespoons fresh mint, chopped
- 1/4 cup grated Parmesan cheese
- Salt and pepper, to taste

Instructions:

1. Preheat the oven to 350ºF (175ºC).
2. In a bowl, whisk together eggs, peas, chopped fresh mint, grated Parmesan cheese, salt, and pepper.
3. Pour egg mixture into a greased oven-safe skillet.
4. Bake for 20-25 minutes or until eggs are set and slightly golden.

5. Slice into wedges and serve hot as a light and refreshing breakfast frittata.

Artichoke and Spinach Breakfast Wrap:

Ingredients:

- 2 large whole grain wraps
- 1 cup baby spinach leaves
- 1/2 cup marinated artichoke hearts, chopped
- 4 large eggs, scrambled
- Salt and pepper, to taste

Instructions:

1. Place whole grain wraps on a flat surface.
2. Divide baby spinach leaves and chopped marinated artichoke hearts evenly between the wraps.
3. Top with scrambled eggs.
4. Season with salt and pepper.
5. Roll up wraps tightly and slice in half.
6. Serve immediately as a Mediterranean-inspired breakfast wrap.

Brussels Sprouts and Bacon Hash:

Ingredients:

- 4 slices bacon, diced
- 2 cups shredded Brussels sprouts
- 1/2 cup diced onions
- Salt and pepper, to taste

Instructions:

1. In a skillet, cook diced bacon over medium heat until crispy.
2. Remove bacon from skillet and set aside.
3. In the same skillet, add shredded Brussels sprouts and diced onions.
4. Cook, stirring occasionally, until Brussels sprouts are tender and onions are translucent.
5. Stir in cooked bacon.
6. Season with salt and pepper.
7. Serve hot as a hearty and indulgent breakfast hash.

Cabbage and Sausage Skillet:

Ingredients:

- 1 tablespoon olive oil
- 1-pound smoked sausage, sliced
- 4 cups shredded cabbage
- 1/2 cup diced onions
- Salt and pepper, to taste

Instructions:

1. Heat olive oil in a large skillet over medium heat.
2. Add sliced smoked sausage and cook until browned.
3. Remove sausage from skillet and set aside.
4. In the same skillet, add shredded cabbage and diced onions.
5. Cook, stirring occasionally, until cabbage is tender and onions are translucent.
6. Stir in cooked sausage.
7. Season with salt and pepper.
8. Serve hot as a comforting and satisfying breakfast skillet.

Green Bean and Tomato Omelet:

Ingredients:

- 6 large eggs
- 1 cup green beans, trimmed and chopped
- 1/2 cup cherry tomatoes, halved
- 1/4 cup shredded mozzarella cheese
- Salt and pepper, to taste

Instructions:

1. In a bowl, whisk together eggs, chopped green beans, halved cherry tomatoes, shredded mozzarella cheese, salt, and pepper.
2. Pour egg mixture into a greased skillet.
3. Cook over medium heat until eggs are set around the edges.
4. Using a spatula, gently lift the edges of the omelet and tilt the skillet to allow the uncooked eggs to flow underneath.
5. Continue cooking until the omelet is set but still slightly moist on top.
6. Fold the omelet in half and slide onto a plate.
7. Serve hot as a colorful and flavorful breakfast option.

Pumpkin and Pecan Smoothie Bowl:

Ingredients:

- 1/2 cup pumpkin puree
- 1 ripe banana
- 1 cup almond milk
- 1/4 teaspoon pumpkin pie spice
- 2 tablespoons chopped pecans
- 1 tablespoon maple syrup

Instructions:

1. In a blender, combine pumpkin puree, ripe banana, almond milk, and pumpkin pie spice.
2. Blend until smooth and creamy.
3. Pour smoothie into a bowl.
4. Top with chopped pecans and a drizzle of maple syrup.
5. Serve immediately as a seasonal and satisfying breakfast smoothie bowl.

Celery and Peanut Butter Toast:

Ingredients:

1. 2 slices whole grain toast
2. 2 tablespoons peanut butter
3. 1 stalk celery, thinly sliced
4. Sprinkle of cinnamon
5. Instructions:
6.
7. Toast whole grain bread until golden brown.
8. Spread peanut butter evenly onto each slice of toast.
9. Arrange thinly sliced celery on top of the peanut butter.
10. Sprinkle it with a dash of cinnamon.
11. Serve immediately as a crunchy and satisfying breakfast option.

Radicchio and Orange Salad:

Ingredients:

1. 2 cups thinly sliced radicchio
2. 1 orange, peeled and segmented
3. 1/4 cup toasted almonds
4. Citrus vinaigrette, for dressing

Instructions:

1. In a large bowl, toss thinly sliced radicchio, orange segments, and toasted almonds.
2. Drizzle with citrus vinaigrette and toss to coat.
3. Serve immediately as a refreshing and vibrant breakfast salad.

Turnip and Chive Scramble:

Ingredients:

- 6 large eggs
- 1 cup diced turnips
- 2 tablespoons fresh chives, chopped
- 1 clove garlic, minced
- 1/4 cup grated Parmesan cheese
- Salt and pepper, to taste

Instructions:

1. In a skillet, sauté diced turnips and minced garlic until tender.
2. In a bowl, whisk together eggs, chopped fresh chives, grated Parmesan cheese, salt, and pepper.
3. Pour egg mixture into the skillet with the cooked turnips.
4. Cook, stirring occasionally, until eggs are scrambled and cooked to desired doneness.
5. Serve hot as a flavorful and satisfying breakfast scramble.

Beet and Goat Cheese Salad:

Ingredients:

- 2 medium beets, roasted and diced
- 2 cups mixed greens
- 1/4 cup walnuts, chopped
- 1/4 cup crumbled goat cheese
- Balsamic vinaigrette, for dressing

Instructions:

1. In a large bowl, toss roasted diced beets, mixed greens, chopped walnuts, and crumbled goat cheese.

2. Drizzle with balsamic vinaigrette and toss to coat.
3. Serve immediately as a colorful and nutrient-rich breakfast salad.

Radish and Avocado Toast:

Ingredients:

- 1 ripe avocado, mashed
- 2 slices whole grain toast
- 4-6 radishes, thinly sliced
- Olive oil, for drizzling

Instructions:

1. Spread mashed avocado evenly onto each slice of whole grain toast.
2. Top with thinly sliced radishes.
3. Drizzle with olive oil.

Serve immediately as a crunchy and refreshing breakfast option

Baked Goods

Banana Oat Muffins:

Ingredients:

- 2 ripe bananas, mashed
- 2 eggs
- 1/4 cup honey or maple syrup
- 1/4 cup coconut oil, melted
- 1 tsp vanilla extract
- 1 1/2 cups old-fashioned oats
- 1 tsp baking powder
- 1/2 tsp baking soda
- 1/2 tsp cinnamon
- 1/4 tsp salt

Instructions:
1. Preheat your oven to 350°F (175°C) and line a muffin tin with paper liners.
2. In a large bowl, whisk together the mashed bananas, eggs, honey or maple syrup, melted coconut oil, and vanilla extract until well combined.
3. In a separate bowl, mix together the oats, baking powder, baking soda, cinnamon, and salt.
4. Gradually add the dry ingredients to the wet ingredients, stirring until just combined.
5. Divide the batter evenly among the muffin cups, filling each about 3/4 full.
6. Bake for 20-25 minutes, or until the muffins are golden brown and a toothpick inserted into the center comes out clean.
7. Allow the muffins to cool in the tin for 5 minutes before transferring them to a wire rack to cool completely. Enjoy!

Blueberry Almond Flour Scones:

Ingredients:

- 2 cups almond flour
- 1/4 cup coconut sugar or honey
- 1/2 tsp baking powder
- 1/4 tsp salt
- 1/4 cup coconut oil, melted
- 1 egg
- 1 tsp vanilla extract
- 1/2 cup fresh or frozen blueberries

Instructions:

1. Preheat your oven to 350°F (175°C) and line a baking sheet with parchment paper.
2. In a large bowl, combine the almond flour, coconut sugar or honey, baking powder, and salt.
3. In a separate bowl, whisk together the melted coconut oil, egg, and vanilla extract.
4. Add the wet ingredients to the dry ingredients and mix until a dough forms.
5. Gently fold in the blueberries until evenly distributed throughout the dough.
6. Transfer the dough to the prepared baking sheet and shape it into a circle about 1 inch thick.
7. Use a knife to cut the dough into 8 wedges, but do not separate them.
8. Bake for 20-25 minutes, or until the scones are golden brown and firm to the touch.
9. Allow the scones to cool on the baking sheet for 5 minutes before transferring them to a wire rack to cool completely. Enjoy warm or at room temperature!

Whole Wheat Banana Bread:

Ingredients:

- 3 ripe bananas, mashed
- 1/3 cup melted coconut oil or butter
- 1/2 cup honey or maple syrup
- 2 eggs
- 1 tsp vanilla extract
- 1 tsp baking soda
- 1/4 tsp salt
- 1 3/4 cups whole wheat flour

Instructions:

1. Preheat your oven to 325°F (165°C) and grease a 9x5-inch loaf pan.
2. In a large bowl, whisk together the mashed bananas, melted coconut oil or butter, honey or maple syrup, eggs, and vanilla extract until well combined.
3. Add the baking soda and salt to the bowl and mix until incorporated.
4. Gradually add the whole wheat flour to the wet ingredients, stirring until just combined.
5. Pour the batter into the prepared loaf pan and smooth the top with a spatula.

6. Bake for 60-70 minutes, or until a toothpick inserted into the center comes out clean.

7. Allow the banana bread to cool in the pan for 10 minutes before transferring it to a wire rack to cool completely. Slice and enjoy!

Pumpkin Spice Loaf with Walnuts:

Ingredients:

- 1 3/4 cups whole wheat flour
- 1 tsp baking soda
- 1/2 tsp baking powder
- 1 tsp ground cinnamon
- 1/2 tsp ground nutmeg
- 1/4 tsp ground cloves
- 1/4 tsp salt
- 2 eggs
- 1 cup pumpkin puree
- 1/2 cup honey or maple syrup
- 1/4 cup melted coconut oil or butter
- 1/2 cup chopped walnuts

Instructions:

1. Preheat your oven to 350°F (175°C) and grease a 9x5-inch loaf pan.

2. In a large bowl, whisk together the whole wheat flour, baking soda, baking powder, cinnamon, nutmeg, cloves, and salt.

3. In a separate bowl, beat the eggs and then add the pumpkin puree, honey or maple syrup, and melted coconut oil or butter. Mix until well combined.

4. Gradually add the wet ingredients to the dry ingredients, stirring until just combined.

5. Fold in the chopped walnuts until evenly distributed throughout the batter.

6. Pour the batter into the prepared loaf pan and smooth the top with a spatula.

7. Bake for 50-60 minutes, or until a toothpick inserted into the center comes out clean.

8. Allow the pumpkin spice loaf to cool in the pan for 10 minutes before transferring it to a wire rack to cool completely. Slice and enjoy!

Zucchini Chocolate Chip Bread:

Ingredients:

- 2 cups grated zucchini
- 1/2 cup coconut sugar or brown sugar
- 1/4 cup melted coconut oil or butter
- 2 eggs
- 1 tsp vanilla extract
- 1 1/2 cups whole wheat flour
- 1 tsp baking powder
- 1/2 tsp baking soda
- 1/2 tsp cinnamon
- 1/4 tsp salt
- 1/2 cup dark chocolate chips

Instructions:

1. Preheat your oven to 350°F (175°C) and grease a 9x5-inch loaf pan.
2. In a large bowl, combine the grated zucchini, coconut sugar or brown sugar, melted coconut oil or butter, eggs, and vanilla extract. Mix until well combined.
3. In a separate bowl, whisk together the whole wheat flour, baking powder, baking soda, cinnamon, and salt.
4. Gradually add the dry ingredients to the wet ingredients, stirring until just combined.
5. Fold in the dark chocolate chips until evenly distributed throughout the batter.
6. Pour the batter into the prepared loaf pan and smooth the top with a spatula.
7. Bake for 50-60 minutes, or until a toothpick inserted into the center comes out clean.
8. Allow the zucchini chocolate chip bread to cool in the pan for 10 minutes before transferring it to a wire rack to cool completely. Slice and enjoy!

Carrot Cake Breakfast Cookies:

Ingredients:

- 2 cups old-fashioned oats
- 1 cup grated carrots
- 1/2 cup chopped walnuts
- 1/4 cup raisins
- 1/4 cup melted coconut oil or butter
- 1/4 cup honey or maple syrup
- 1 egg
- 1 tsp vanilla extract
- 1 tsp ground cinnamon
- 1/4 tsp ground nutmeg

- 1/4 tsp salt

Instructions:

1. Preheat your oven to 350°F (175°C) and line a baking sheet with parchment paper.
2. In a large bowl, combine the oats, grated carrots, chopped walnuts, and raisins.
3. In a separate bowl, whisk together the melted coconut oil or butter, honey or maple syrup, egg, vanilla extract, cinnamon, nutmeg, and salt.
4. Pour the wet ingredients into the dry ingredients and mix until well combined.
5. Use a cookie scoop or spoon to drop the dough onto the prepared baking sheet, spacing the cookies about 2 inches apart.
6. Flatten each cookie slightly with the back of a spoon.
7. Bake for 12-15 minutes, or until the cookies are golden brown around the edges.
8. Allow the carrot cake breakfast cookies to cool on the baking sheet for 5 minutes before transferring them to a wire rack to cool completely. Enjoy!

Lemon Poppy Seed Loaf:

Ingredients:

- 1 1/2 cups almond flour
- 1/4 cup coconut flour
- 1/4 cup coconut sugar or honey
- 1 tsp baking powder
- 1/2 tsp baking soda
- 1/4 tsp salt
- 1/4 cup melted coconut oil or butter
- 1/4 cup lemon juice
- 2 eggs
- 1 tsp vanilla extract
- Zest of 1 lemon
- 1 tbsp poppy seeds

Instructions:

1. Preheat your oven to 350°F (175°C) and grease a 9x5-inch loaf pan.
2. In a large bowl, whisk together the almond flour, coconut flour, coconut sugar or honey, baking powder, baking soda, and salt.
3. In a separate bowl, whisk together the melted coconut oil or butter, lemon juice, eggs, vanilla extract, and lemon zest.
4. Gradually add the wet ingredients to the dry ingredients, stirring until well combined.

5. Fold in the poppy seeds until evenly distributed throughout the batter.
6. Pour the batter into the prepared loaf pan and smooth the top with a spatula.
7. Bake for 40-45 minutes, or until a toothpick inserted into the center comes out clean.
8. Allow the lemon poppy seed loaf to cool in the pan for 10 minutes before transferring it to a wire rack to cool completely. Slice and enjoy!

Apple Cinnamon Muffins:

Ingredients:

- 2 cups whole wheat flour
- 1/2 cup coconut sugar or brown sugar
- 2 tsp baking powder
- 1/2 tsp baking soda
- 1/2 tsp cinnamon
- 1/4 tsp salt
- 2 eggs
- 1/4 cup melted coconut oil or butter
- 1/2 cup unsweetened applesauce
- 1/2 cup almond milk or other milk of choice
- 1 tsp vanilla extract
- 1 apple, peeled and diced

Instructions:

1. Preheat your oven to 375°F (190°C) and line a muffin tin with paper liners.
2. In a large bowl, whisk together the whole wheat flour, coconut sugar or brown sugar, baking powder, baking soda, cinnamon, and salt.
3. In a separate bowl, beat the eggs and then add the melted coconut oil or butter, applesauce, almond milk, and vanilla extract. Mix until well combined.
4. Gradually add the wet ingredients to the dry ingredients, stirring until just combined.
5. Gently fold in the diced apple until evenly distributed throughout the batter.
6. Divide the batter evenly among the muffin cups, filling each about 3/4 full.
7. Bake for 18-20 minutes, or until the muffins are golden brown and a toothpick inserted into the center comes out clean.
8. Allow the apple cinnamon muffins to cool in the tin for 5

minutes before transferring them to a wire rack to cool completely. Enjoy!

Coconut Flour Pancakes:

Ingredients:

- 1/2 cup coconut flour
- 4 eggs
- 1/2 cup almond milk or other milk of choice
- 2 tbsp melted coconut oil or butter
- 1 tbsp honey or maple syrup
- 1 tsp vanilla extract
- 1/2 tsp baking powder
- 1/4 tsp salt

Instructions:

1. In a large bowl, whisk together the coconut flour, eggs, almond milk, melted coconut oil or butter, honey or maple syrup, vanilla extract, baking powder, and salt until well combined.
2. Let the batter sit for a few minutes to allow the coconut flour to absorb the liquid.
3. Heat a non-stick skillet or griddle over medium heat and lightly grease with coconut oil or butter.
4. Pour about 1/4 cup of batter onto the skillet for each pancake, spreading it out slightly with the back of a spoon.
5. Cook for 2-3 minutes, or until bubbles form on the surface of the pancake and the edges begin to set.
6. Flip the pancakes and cook for another 1-2 minutes, or until golden brown on the bottom.
7. Repeat with the remaining batter, greasing the skillet as needed.
8. Serve the coconut flour pancakes warm with your favorite toppings, such as fresh fruit, maple syrup, or nut butter. Enjoy!

Almond Butter Banana Bars:

Ingredients:

- 2 ripe bananas, mashed
- 1/2 cup almond butter
- 1/4 cup honey or maple syrup
- 2 eggs
- 1 tsp vanilla extract
- 1 1/2 cups almond flour
- 1/2 tsp baking soda
- 1/4 tsp salt

- 1/2 cup dark chocolate chips (optional)

Instructions:

1. Preheat your oven to 350°F (175°C) and grease an 8x8-inch baking dish.
2. In a large bowl, whisk together the mashed bananas, almond butter, honey or maple syrup, eggs, and vanilla extract until well combined.
3. In a separate bowl, combine the almond flour, baking soda, and salt.
4. Gradually add the dry ingredients to the wet ingredients, stirring until just combined.
5. Fold in the dark chocolate chips, if using.
6. Pour the batter into the prepared baking dish and smooth the top with a spatula.
7. Bake for 20-25 minutes, or until the bars are golden brown and set in the center.
8. Allow the almond butter banana bars to cool in the dish for 10 minutes before slicing into squares. Enjoy as a snack or breakfast on the go!

Quinoa Breakfast Bars:

Ingredients:

- 1 cup cooked quinoa
- 1/2 cup almond butter
- 1/4 cup honey or maple syrup
- 1 egg
- 1 tsp vanilla extract
- 1/2 tsp cinnamon
- 1/4 tsp salt
- 1/4 cup chopped nuts (such as almonds, walnuts, or pecans)
- 1/4 cup dried fruit (such as raisins, cranberries, or chopped apricots)
- 1/4 cup shredded coconut (optional)

Instructions:

1. Preheat your oven to 350°F (175°C) and line an 8x8-inch baking dish with parchment paper.
2. In a large bowl, mix together the cooked quinoa, almond butter, honey or maple syrup, egg, vanilla extract, cinnamon, and salt until well combined.
3. Stir in the chopped nuts, dried fruit, and shredded coconut, if using.
4. Press the mixture into the prepared baking dish,

smoothing the top with a spatula.

5. Bake for 20-25 minutes, or until the bars are golden brown and set in the center.

6. Allow the quinoa breakfast bars to cool in the dish for 10 minutes before slicing into squares. Enjoy as a nutritious and portable breakfast option!

Cranberry Orange Scones:

Ingredients:

- 2 cups almond flour
- 1/4 cup coconut flour
- 1/4 cup coconut sugar or honey
- 1 tsp baking powder
- 1/4 tsp baking soda
- 1/4 tsp salt
- Zest of 1 orange
- 1/4 cup coconut oil, solid
- 1/4 cup freshly squeezed orange juice
- 1 egg
- 1/2 cup dried cranberries

Instructions:

1. Preheat your oven to 350°F (175°C) and line a baking sheet with parchment paper.

2. In a large bowl, whisk together the almond flour, coconut flour, coconut sugar or honey, baking powder, baking soda, salt, and orange zest.

3. Add the solid coconut oil to the bowl and use your fingers or a pastry cutter to work it into the dry ingredients until the mixture resembles coarse crumbs.

4. In a separate bowl, whisk together the orange juice and egg.

5. Gradually add the wet ingredients to the dry ingredients, stirring until a dough forms.

6. Gently fold in the dried cranberries until evenly distributed throughout the dough.

7. Transfer the dough to the prepared baking sheet and shape it into a circle about 1 inch thick.

8. Use a knife to cut the dough into 8 wedges, but do not separate them.

9. Bake for 18-20 minutes, or until the scones are golden brown and firm to the touch.

10. Allow the cranberry orange scones to cool on the baking sheet for 5 minutes before transferring them to a wire rack

to cool completely. Enjoy warm or at room temperature!

Sweet Potato Biscuits:

Ingredients:

- 1 cup mashed sweet potato (from about 2 small sweet potatoes)
- 1/4 cup melted coconut oil or butter
- 1/4 cup almond milk or other milk of choice
- 2 tbsp honey or maple syrup
- 2 cups whole wheat flour
- 1 tbsp baking powder
- 1/2 tsp salt

Instructions:

1. Preheat your oven to 425°F (220°C) and line a baking sheet with parchment paper.
2. In a large bowl, whisk together the mashed sweet potato, melted coconut oil or butter, almond milk, and honey or maple syrup until well combined.
3. In a separate bowl, combine the whole wheat flour, baking powder, and salt.
4. Gradually add the dry ingredients to the wet ingredients, stirring until just combined.
5. Turn the dough out onto a lightly floured surface and knead it gently a few times until it comes together.
6. Roll out the dough to about 1/2-inch thickness and use a biscuit cutter to cut out biscuits.
7. Place the biscuits on the prepared baking sheet and bake for 12-15 minutes, or until golden brown.
8. Allow the sweet potato biscuits to cool on the baking sheet for a few minutes before transferring them to a wire rack to cool completely. Enjoy warm with a drizzle of honey or a pat of butter!

Gingerbread Muffins:

Ingredients:

- 2 cups whole wheat flour
- 1/2 cup coconut sugar or brown sugar
- 1 tsp baking powder
- 1/2 tsp baking soda
- 1 tsp ground ginger
- 1/2 tsp ground cinnamon

- 1/4 tsp ground cloves
- 1/4 tsp salt
- 2 eggs
- 1/4 cup molasses
- 1/4 cup melted coconut oil or butter
- 1/2 cup almond milk or other milk of choice
- 1 tsp vanilla extract

Instructions:

1. Preheat your oven to 350ºF (175ºC) and line a muffin tin with paper liners.
2. In a large bowl, whisk together the whole wheat flour, coconut sugar or brown sugar, baking powder, baking soda, ginger, cinnamon, cloves, and salt.
3. In a separate bowl, beat the eggs and then add the molasses, melted coconut oil or butter, almond milk, and vanilla extract. Mix until well combined.
4. Gradually add the wet ingredients to the dry ingredients, stirring until just combined.
5. Divide the batter evenly among the muffin cups, filling each about 3/4 full.
6. Bake for 18-20 minutes, or until the muffins are golden brown and a toothpick inserted into the center comes out clean.
7. Allow the gingerbread muffins to cool in the tin for 5 minutes before transferring them to a wire rack to cool completely. Enjoy warm or at room temperature!

Raspberry Oatmeal Bars:

Ingredients:

- 1 cup rolled oats
- 1 cup whole wheat flour
- 1/2 cup almond flour
- 1/2 cup coconut sugar
- 1/2 teaspoon baking powder
- 1/4 teaspoon salt
- 1/2 cup coconut oil, melted
- 1/4 cup maple syrup
- 1 teaspoon vanilla extract
- 1 cup fresh raspberries

Instructions:

1. Preheat the oven to 350ºF (175ºC). Grease or line a baking dish with parchment paper.
2. In a large bowl, combine the rolled oats, whole wheat flour, almond flour, coconut sugar, baking powder, and salt.

3. Add the melted coconut oil, maple syrup, and vanilla extract to the dry ingredients. Mix until well combined.
4. Press half of the mixture into the bottom of the prepared baking dish.
5. Spread the raspberries evenly over the oat mixture.
6. Sprinkle the remaining oat mixture over the raspberries, pressing down lightly.
7. Bake for 25-30 minutes, or until golden brown.
8. Allow to cool completely before slicing into bars. Enjoy!

Chia Seed Breakfast Cookies:

Ingredients:
- 2 ripe bananas, mashed
- 1/4 cup almond butter
- 1/4 cup maple syrup
- 1 teaspoon vanilla extract
- 1 cup rolled oats
- 1/4 cup chia seeds
- 1/4 cup dried cranberries
- 1/4 cup chopped walnuts (optional)

Instructions:

1. Preheat the oven to 350°F (175°C). Line a baking sheet with parchment paper.
2. In a large bowl, combine the mashed bananas, almond butter, maple syrup, and vanilla extract.
3. Stir in the rolled oats, chia seeds, dried cranberries, and chopped walnuts until well combined.
4. Drop spoonful of the cookie dough onto the prepared baking sheet, spacing them apart.
5. Flatten each cookie slightly with the back of a spoon.
6. Bake for 12-15 minutes, or until golden brown.
7. Allow to cool on the baking sheet for 5 minutes before transferring to a wire rack to cool completely. Enjoy as a nutritious breakfast or snack on the go!

Spinach and Feta Breakfast Muffins:

Ingredients:

- 2 cups whole wheat flour
- 1 tablespoon baking powder
- 1/2 teaspoon salt

- 1/4 teaspoon black pepper
- 2 eggs
- 1 cup milk
- 1/4 cup olive oil
- 1 cup chopped spinach
- 1/2 cup crumbled feta cheese

Instructions:

1. Preheat the oven to 375°F (190°C). Grease a muffin tin or line with paper liners.
2. In a large bowl, whisk together the whole wheat flour, baking powder, salt, and black pepper.
3. In a separate bowl, beat the eggs, then stir in the milk and olive oil.
4. Pour the wet ingredients into the dry ingredients and mix until just combined.
5. Fold in the chopped spinach and crumbled feta cheese.
6. Divide the batter evenly among the prepared muffin cups.
7. Bake for 20-25 minutes, or until the muffins are golden brown and a toothpick inserted into the center comes out clean.
8. Allow the muffins to cool in the tin for 5 minutes before transferring to a wire rack to cool completely. Enjoy warm or at room temperature!

Peach Streusel Coffee Cake:

Ingredients:

- 2 cups whole wheat flour
- 1 teaspoon baking powder
- 1/2 teaspoon baking soda
- 1/4 teaspoon salt
- 1/2 cup unsweetened applesauce
- 1/4 cup coconut oil, melted
- 1/2 cup maple syrup
- 1/4 cup almond milk
- 2 teaspoons vanilla extract
- 2 cups diced peaches (fresh or canned, drained)
- Streusel Topping:
- 1/4 cup whole wheat flour
- 1/4 cup rolled oats
- 1/4 cup coconut sugar
- 2 tablespoons coconut oil, melted
- 1/2 teaspoon cinnamon

Instructions:

1. Preheat the oven to 350°F (175°C). Grease a 9x9-inch baking dish.
2. In a large bowl, whisk together the whole wheat flour, baking powder, baking soda, and salt.

3. In a separate bowl, combine the applesauce, melted coconut oil, maple syrup, almond milk, and vanilla extract.
4. Pour the wet ingredients into the dry ingredients and mix until just combined.
5. Gently fold in the diced peaches.
6. Pour the batter into the prepared baking dish, spreading it out evenly.
7. In a small bowl, combine the streusel topping ingredients until crumbly.
8. Sprinkle the streusel topping evenly over the batter.
9. Bake for 30-35 minutes, or until a toothpick inserted into the center comes out clean.
10. Allow the coffee cake to cool in the pan for 10 minutes before slicing and serving. Enjoy with a cup of coffee or tea for a delightful breakfast or snack!

Chocolate Avocado Brownies:

Ingredients:
- 2 ripe avocados
- 1/2 cup maple syrup
- 1/4 cup cocoa powder
- 2 eggs
- 1 teaspoon vanilla extract
- 1/2 cup whole wheat flour
- 1/4 teaspoon salt
- 1/2 cup dark chocolate chips

Instructions:
1. Preheat the oven to 350°F (175°C). Grease or line a baking dish with parchment paper.
2. In a food processor, blend the avocados until smooth.
3. Add the maple syrup, cocoa powder, eggs, and vanilla extract to the avocado puree. Blend until well combined.
4. Transfer the mixture to a mixing bowl and fold in the whole wheat flour and salt until just combined.
5. Fold in the dark chocolate chips.
6. Pour the batter into the prepared baking dish and spread it out evenly.
7. Bake for 25-30 minutes, or until the edges are set and a toothpick inserted into the center comes out mostly clean.
8. Allow the brownies to cool completely before slicing into squares. Enjoy these fudgy, indulgent treats guilt-free!

Cinnamon Raisin Bagels:

Ingredients:
- 1 cup warm water
- 2 1/4 teaspoons active dry yeast
- 2 tablespoons coconut sugar
- 3 cups whole wheat flour
- 1 teaspoon salt
- 1 teaspoon ground cinnamon
- 1/2 cup raisins

Instructions:
1. In a small bowl, combine the warm water, active dry yeast, and coconut sugar. Let it sit for 5 minutes until frothy.
2. In a large mixing bowl, combine the whole wheat flour, salt, and ground cinnamon.
3. Pour the yeast mixture into the dry ingredients and mix until a dough forms.
4. Knead the dough on a lightly floured surface for 5-7 minutes, or until smooth and elastic.
5. Flatten the dough and sprinkle the raisins evenly over the surface. Fold the dough over the raisins and knead gently to distribute them throughout.
6. Divide the dough into 6 equal portions and shape each portion into a smooth ball.
7. Use your finger to poke a hole through the center of each dough ball, then gently stretch the hole to form a bagel shape.
8. Place the shaped bagels on a baking sheet lined with parchment paper and cover with a clean kitchen towel. Let them rise in a warm place for 30-45 minutes.
9. Preheat the oven to 375°F (190°C).
10. Bring a large pot of water to a boil. Boil the bagels, 2-3 at a time, for 1-2 minutes on each side.
11. Remove the boiled bagels from the water and place them back on the baking sheet.
12. Bake the bagels for 20-25 minutes, or until golden brown and cooked through.
13. Allow the bagels to cool on a wire rack before slicing and enjoying with your favorite toppings. These homemade bagels are perfect for a satisfying breakfast or snack!

Honey Oat Bread:

Ingredients:

- 1 cup warm water
- 2 1/4 teaspoons active dry yeast
- 2 tablespoons honey
- 2 tablespoons olive oil
- 2 cups whole wheat flour
- 1 cup rolled oats
- 1 teaspoon salt

Instructions:

1. In a small bowl, combine the warm water, active dry yeast, and honey. Let it sit for 5 minutes until frothy.
2. In a large mixing bowl, combine the whole wheat flour, rolled oats, and salt.
3. Pour the yeast mixture and olive oil into the dry ingredients and mix until a dough forms.
4. Knead the dough on a lightly floured surface for 5-7 minutes, or until smooth and elastic.
5. Shape the dough into a loaf and place it in a greased loaf pan.
6. Cover the loaf pan with a clean kitchen towel and let the dough rise in a warm place for 30-45 minutes, or until doubled in size.
7. Preheat the oven to 375°F (190°C).
8. Bake the bread for 30-35 minutes, or until golden brown and hollow-sounding when tapped on the bottom.
9. Remove the bread from the oven and let it cool in the pan for 5 minutes before transferring to a wire rack to cool completely. Enjoy slices of this hearty honey oat bread toasted with your favorite toppings for a nutritious breakfast or snack!

Almond Flour Pancakes with Berries:

Ingredients:

- 1 cup almond flour
- 2 tablespoons coconut flour
- 1 teaspoon baking powder
- 1/4 teaspoon salt
- 2 eggs
- 1/4 cup almond milk
- 2 tablespoons maple syrup
- 1 teaspoon vanilla extract
- Fresh berries, for serving
- Maple syrup, for serving

Instructions:

1. In a large mixing bowl, whisk together the almond flour, coconut flour, baking powder, and salt.

2. In a separate bowl, whisk together the eggs, almond milk, maple syrup, and vanilla extract.

3. Pour the wet ingredients into the dry ingredients and mix until smooth.

4. Heat a non-stick skillet or griddle over medium heat and lightly grease with coconut oil or cooking spray.

5. Pour about 1/4 cup of batter onto the skillet for each pancake.

6. Cook the pancakes for 2-3 minutes on one side, until bubbles form on the surface.

7. Flip the pancakes and cook for an additional 1-2 minutes on the other side, until golden brown and cooked through.

8. Serve the pancakes warm with fresh berries and maple syrup. Enjoy these fluffy almond flour pancakes as a delicious and filling breakfast option!

Whole Grain Fig Bars:

Ingredients:
- 1/2 cups whole wheat flour
- 1/2 cup rolled oats
- 1/2 cup coconut sugar
- 1/2 teaspoon baking powder
- 1/4 teaspoon salt
- 1/2 cup coconut oil, melted
- 1/4 cup almond milk
- 1 teaspoon vanilla extract
- 1 cup fig jam or preserves

Instructions:

1. Preheat the oven to 350°F (175°C). Grease or line a baking dish with parchment paper.

2. In a large bowl, combine the whole wheat flour, rolled oats, coconut sugar, baking powder, and salt.

3. Stir in the melted coconut oil, almond milk, and vanilla extract until a dough forms.

4. Press half of the dough into the bottom of the prepared baking dish, creating an even layer.

5. Spread the fig jam evenly over the dough layer.

6. Crumble the remaining dough over the fig jam layer, covering it completely.

7. Bake for 25-30 minutes, or until the top is golden brown.

8. Allow to cool completely before slicing into bars. Enjoy these wholesome fig bars as a satisfying snack or dessert option!

Pecan Date Bread:

Ingredients:

- 1 cup whole wheat flour
- 1 teaspoon baking powder
- 1/2 teaspoon baking soda
- 1/4 teaspoon salt
- 1 cup mashed ripe bananas
- 1/4 cup maple syrup
- 1/4 cup coconut oil, melted
- 2 eggs
- 1 teaspoon vanilla extract
- 1/2 cup chopped dates
- 1/2 cup chopped pecans

Instructions:

1. Preheat the oven to 350ºF (175ºC). Grease or line a loaf pan with parchment paper.
2. In a large bowl, whisk together the whole wheat flour, baking powder, baking soda, and salt.
3. In a separate bowl, combine the mashed bananas, maple syrup, melted coconut oil, eggs, and vanilla extract.
4. Pour the wet ingredients into the dry ingredients and mix until just combined.
5. Fold in the chopped dates and chopped pecans until evenly distributed.
6. Pour the batter into the prepared loaf pan and spread it out evenly.
7. Bake for 45-50 minutes, or until a toothpick inserted into the center comes out clean.
8. Allow the bread to cool in the pan for 10 minutes before transferring to a wire rack to cool completely. Slice and enjoy this moist and flavorful pecan date bread for breakfast or as a snack!

Blueberry Cornmeal Muffins:

Ingredients:

1. 1 cup cornmeal
2. 1 cup whole wheat flour
3. 1/4 cup coconut sugar
4. 1 tablespoon baking powder
5. 1/2 teaspoon salt
6. 1 cup almond milk
7. 1/4 cup coconut oil, melted
8. 2 eggs
9. 1 teaspoon vanilla extract
10. 1 cup fresh or frozen blueberries

Instructions:

1. Preheat the oven to 375ºF (190ºC). Grease a muffin tin or line with paper liners.
2. In a large bowl, whisk together the cornmeal, whole wheat flour, coconut sugar, baking powder, and salt.

3. In a separate bowl, mix together the almond milk, melted coconut oil, eggs, and vanilla extract until well combined.
4. Pour the wet ingredients into the dry ingredients and stir until just combined. Be careful not to overmix.
5. Gently fold in the blueberries.
6. Divide the batter evenly among the prepared muffin cups.
7. Bake for 20-25 minutes, or until a toothpick inserted into the center of a muffin comes out clean.
8. Allow the muffins to cool in the tin for a few minutes before transferring them to a wire rack to cool completely. Enjoy these tender and flavorful blueberry cornmeal muffins for breakfast or as a snack!

Coconut Almond Granola Bars:

Ingredients:

- 2 cups rolled oats
- 1/2 cup shredded coconut
- 1/2 cup chopped almonds
- 1/4 cup coconut oil, melted
- 1/4 cup honey
- 1 teaspoon vanilla extract
- 1/4 teaspoon salt
- 1/2 cup dried cranberries (optional)

Instructions:

1. Preheat the oven to 350°F (175°C). Line a baking dish with parchment paper, leaving some overhang on the sides for easy removal.
2. In a large bowl, combine the rolled oats, shredded coconut, chopped almonds, and salt.
3. In a separate bowl, mix together the melted coconut oil, honey, and vanilla extract.
4. Pour the wet ingredients over the dry ingredients and stir until everything is well coated.
5. Press the mixture firmly and evenly into the prepared baking dish.
6. Bake for 20-25 minutes, or until the edges are golden brown.
7. Allow the granola bars to cool completely in the baking dish.
8. Once cooled, use the parchment paper overhang to lift the bars out of the dish. Cut into bars or squares.
9. Store the granola bars in an airtight container at room temperature for up to a week. Enjoy these homemade coconut almond granola bars as a

nutritious and satisfying snack on the go!

Spinach and Cheese Breakfast Casserole.

Ingredients:
- 6 slices whole grain bread, cubed
- 1 cup chopped spinach, fresh or frozen (thawed and drained)
- 1 cup shredded cheddar cheese
- 6 eggs
- 1 cup almond milk
- 1 teaspoon Dijon mustard
- 1/2 teaspoon garlic powder
- Salt and pepper to taste

Instructions:
1. Preheat the oven to 350°F (175°C). Grease a 9x13-inch baking dish.
2. Spread the cubed bread evenly in the prepared baking dish.
3. Sprinkle the chopped spinach and shredded cheddar cheese over the bread cubes.
4. In a large bowl, whisk together the eggs, almond milk, Dijon mustard, garlic powder, salt, and pepper.
5. Pour the egg mixture evenly over the bread, spinach, and cheese in the baking dish.
6. Gently press down on the bread mixture with a spatula to ensure that it is evenly soaked in the egg mixture.
7. Cover the baking dish with foil and bake for 30 minutes.
8. Remove the foil and bake for an additional 15-20 minutes, or until the top is golden brown and the eggs are set.
9. Allow the breakfast casserole to cool for a few minutes before slicing and serving. Enjoy this hearty and flavorful dish for breakfast or brunch!

Orange Cranberry Biscotti:

Ingredients:
- 2 cups whole wheat flour
- 1/2 cup coconut sugar
- 1 teaspoon baking powder
- Zest of 1 orange
- 1/2 cup fresh orange juice
- 2 eggs
- 1 teaspoon vanilla extract
- 1/2 cup dried cranberries
- 1/2 cup chopped almonds

Instructions:

1. Preheat the oven to 350°F (175°C). Line a baking sheet with parchment paper.
2. In a large bowl, whisk together the whole wheat flour, coconut sugar, baking powder, and orange zest.
3. In a separate bowl, whisk together the fresh orange juice, eggs, and vanilla extract.
4. Pour the wet ingredients into the dry ingredients and stir until a dough forms.
5. Fold in the dried cranberries and chopped almonds until evenly distributed.
6. Divide the dough in half and shape each half into a log on the prepared baking sheet.
7. Bake for 25-30 minutes, or until the logs are firm and lightly golden.
8. Remove the biscotti logs from the oven and let them cool for 10 minutes.
9. Reduce the oven temperature to 325°F (160°C).
10. Carefully slice the logs into diagonal slices using a serrated knife.
11. Place the sliced biscotti back on the baking sheet and bake for an additional 10-15 minutes, or until crisp and golden.
12. Allow the biscotti to cool completely before enjoying it with a cup of tea or coffee. These orange cranberry biscotti make a delightful and flavorful treat!

Raspberry Coconut Muffins:

Ingredients:

- 1/2 cups whole wheat flour
- 1/2 cup coconut sugar
- 1 teaspoon baking powder
- 1/2 teaspoon baking soda
- 1/4 teaspoon salt
- 1 cup unsweetened coconut milk
- 1/4 cup coconut oil, melted
- 1 teaspoon vanilla extract
- 1 cup fresh raspberries

Instructions:

1. Preheat the oven to 375°F (190°C). Grease a muffin tin or line with paper liners.
2. In a large bowl, whisk together the whole wheat flour, coconut sugar, baking powder, baking soda, and salt.
3. In a separate bowl, mix together the coconut milk, melted coconut oil, and vanilla extract.
4. Pour the wet ingredients into the dry ingredients and stir until just combined.

5. Gently fold in the fresh raspberries.
6. Divide the batter evenly among the prepared muffin cups.
7. Bake for 20-25 minutes, or until a toothpick inserted into the center of a muffin comes out clean.
8. Allow the muffins to cool in the tin for a few minutes before transferring them to a wire rack to cool completely. Enjoy these moist and fruity raspberry coconut muffins for breakfast or as a snack!

Apricot Almond Biscuits:

Ingredients:
- 1/2 cups whole wheat flour
- 1/2 cup almond flour
- 1/4 cup coconut sugar
- 1 tablespoon baking powder
- 1/4 teaspoon salt
- 1/2 cup unsweetened almond milk
- 1/4 cup coconut oil, melted
- 1 teaspoon almond extract
- 1/2 cup chopped dried apricots
- 1/4 cup sliced almonds

Instructions:
1. Preheat the oven to 375°F (190°C). Line a baking sheet with parchment paper.
2. In a large bowl, whisk together the whole wheat flour, almond flour, coconut sugar, baking powder, and salt.
3. In a separate bowl, mix together the almond milk, melted coconut oil, and almond extract.
4. Pour the wet ingredients into the dry ingredients and stir until just combined.
5. Gently fold in the chopped dried apricots.
6. Drop spoonful of the biscuit dough onto the prepared baking sheet, spacing them apart.
7. Press a few sliced almonds onto the top of each biscuit.
8. Bake for 12-15 minutes, or until the biscuits are golden brown and cooked through.
9. Allow the biscuits to cool on the baking sheet for 5 minutes before transferring them to a wire rack to cool completely. Enjoy these tender and flavorful apricot almond biscuits with a cup of tea or coffee!

Cherry Vanilla Scones:

Ingredients:
- 2 cups whole wheat flour
- 1/4 cup coconut sugar

- 1 tablespoon baking powder
- 1/4 teaspoon salt
- 1/2 cup coconut oil, solid
- 1/2 cup unsweetened almond milk
- 1 teaspoon vanilla extract
- 1/2 cup chopped fresh or frozen cherries

Instructions:

1. Preheat the oven to 400°F (200°C). Line a baking sheet with parchment paper.
2. In a large bowl, whisk together the whole wheat flour, coconut sugar, baking powder, and salt.
3. Cut the solid coconut oil into the flour mixture using a pastry cutter or fork until it resembles coarse crumbs.
4. In a small bowl, mix together the almond milk and vanilla extract.
5. Gradually pour the almond milk mixture into the flour mixture, stirring until a dough forms.
6. Gently fold in the chopped cherries until evenly distributed.
7. Transfer the dough onto a lightly floured surface and shape it into a circle about 1 inch thick.
8. Use a knife to cut the circle into 8 wedges.
9. Place the scones on the prepared baking sheet and bake for 15-18 minutes, or until golden brown.
10. Allow the scones to cool on the baking sheet for a few minutes before transferring them to a wire rack to cool completely. Enjoy these cherry vanilla scones warm or at room temperature with a cup of tea or coffee!

Egg Recipes

Veggie Egg Scramble:

Ingredients:

- 4 eggs
- 1/4 cup diced bell peppers
- 1/4 cup diced onions
- 1/4 cup diced tomatoes
- 1/4 cup chopped spinach
- Salt and pepper to taste
- 1 tablespoon olive oil

Instructions:

1. Heat olive oil in a non-stick skillet over medium heat.
2. Add diced bell peppers and onions to the skillet and sauté until softened, about 2-3 minutes.
3. Add diced tomatoes and chopped spinach to the skillet and cook until spinach is wilted, about 1-2 minutes.
4. In a bowl, beat the eggs and season with salt and pepper.
5. Pour the beaten eggs into the skillet with the veggies.
6. Cook, stirring occasionally, until the eggs are scrambled and cooked through, about 3-4 minutes.
7. Serve hot and enjoy!

Spinach and Feta Omelet:

Ingredients:

- 3 eggs
- 1/4 cup chopped spinach
- 2 tablespoons crumbled feta cheese
- Salt and pepper to taste
- 1 teaspoon olive oil

Instructions:

In a bowl, beat the eggs and season with salt and pepper.

Heat olive oil in a non-stick skillet over medium heat.

Pour the beaten eggs into the skillet and swirl to coat the bottom evenly.

Cook for 1-2 minutes until the edges begin to set.

Sprinkle chopped spinach and crumbled feta cheese over one half of the omelet.

Carefully fold the other half of the omelet over the filling.

Cook for another 1-2 minutes until the cheese is melted and the omelet is cooked through. Slide onto a plate, cut in half, and serve hot.

Mushroom and Swiss Cheese Frittata:

Ingredients:

- 6 eggs
- 1 cup sliced mushrooms
- 1/2 cup shredded Swiss cheese
- Salt and pepper to taste
- 1 tablespoon olive oil

Instructions:

1. Preheat the oven to 350°F (175°C).
2. In a mixing bowl, beat the eggs and season with salt and pepper.
3. Heat olive oil in an oven-safe skillet over medium heat.
4. Add sliced mushrooms to the skillet and sauté until softened, about 3-4 minutes.
5. Pour the beaten eggs into the skillet over the mushrooms.
6. Sprinkle shredded Swiss cheese evenly over the eggs.
7. Transfer the skillet to the preheated oven and bake for 12-

15 minutes, or until the eggs are set and the cheese is melted and bubbly.

8. Remove from the oven, slice into wedges, and serve hot.

Tomato Basil Egg Cups:

Ingredients:

- 6 eggs
- 1/2 cup diced tomatoes
- 1/4 cup chopped fresh basil
- Salt and pepper to taste
- Cooking spray

Instructions:

1. Preheat the oven to 375°F (190°C) and lightly grease a muffin tin with cooking spray.
2. Crack an egg into each muffin cup.
3. Divide diced tomatoes and chopped fresh basil evenly among the muffin cups.
4. Season each egg cup with salt and pepper to taste.
5. Bake in the preheated oven for 12-15 minutes, or until the eggs are set to your desired level of doneness.

6. Remove from the oven, let cool slightly, and carefully remove the egg cups from the muffin tin.
7. Serve warm and enjoy!

Mediterranean Egg Bake:

Ingredients:

- 8 eggs
- 1/2 cup diced bell peppers
- 1/2 cup diced red onions
- 1/2 cup diced tomatoes
- 1/4 cup chopped kalamata olives
- 1/4 cup crumbled feta cheese
- 2 tablespoons chopped fresh parsley
- Salt and pepper to taste
- Cooking spray

Instructions:

1. Preheat the oven to 375°F (190°C) and lightly grease a baking dish with cooking spray.
2. In a mixing bowl, beat the eggs and season with salt and pepper.
3. Spread diced bell peppers, red onions, tomatoes, and kalamata olives evenly in the prepared baking dish.
4. Pour the beaten eggs over the vegetables in the baking dish.
5. Sprinkle crumbled feta cheese and chopped fresh parsley over the eggs.
6. Bake in the preheated oven for 25-30 minutes, or until the eggs are set and the top is golden brown.
7. Remove from the oven, let cool slightly, and slice into squares.
8. Serve warm and enjoy!

Broccoli and Cheddar Quiche:

Ingredients:

- 1 pie crust (store-bought or homemade)
- 4 eggs
- 1 cup chopped broccoli florets
- 1 cup shredded cheddar cheese
- 1/2 cup milk or cream
- Salt and pepper to taste
- Cooking spray

Instructions:

1. Preheat the oven to 375°F (190°C) and place the pie crust in a pie dish, pressing it firmly into the bottom and sides.

2. In a mixing bowl, beat the eggs and whisk in the milk or cream until well combined.
3. Spread chopped broccoli florets and shredded cheddar cheese evenly in the prepared pie crust.
4. Pour the egg mixture over the broccoli and cheese.
5. Season with salt and pepper to taste.
6. Bake in the preheated oven for 35-40 minutes, or until the filling is set and the top is golden brown.
7. Remove from the oven, let cool slightly, and slice into wedges.
8. Serve warm or at room temperature, and enjoy!

Asparagus and Goat Cheese Frittata:

Ingredients:

- 6 eggs
- 1/2 cup chopped asparagus
- 1/4 cup crumbled goat cheese
- 2 tablespoons chopped fresh chives
- Salt and pepper to taste
- 1 tablespoon olive oil

Instructions:

1. Preheat the oven to 375°F (190°C).
2. In a mixing bowl, beat the eggs and season with salt and pepper.
3. Heat olive oil in an oven-safe skillet over medium heat.
4. Add chopped asparagus to the skillet and sauté until tender, about 4-5 minutes.
5. Pour the beaten eggs into the skillet over the asparagus.
6. Sprinkle crumbled goat cheese and chopped fresh chives evenly over the eggs.
7. Transfer the skillet to the preheated oven and bake for 12-15 minutes, or until the eggs are set and the top is golden brown.
8. Remove from the oven, slice into wedges, and serve hot.

Smoked Salmon and Dill Egg Muffins:

Ingredients:

- 6 eggs
- 1/4 cup chopped smoked salmon
- 2 tablespoons chopped fresh dill
- Salt and pepper to taste
- Cooking spray

Instructions:

1. Preheat the oven to 375ºF (190ºC) and lightly grease a muffin tin with cooking spray.
2. Crack an egg into each muffin cup.
3. Divide chopped smoked salmon and chopped fresh dill evenly among the muffin cups.
4. Season each egg cup with salt and pepper to taste.
5. Bake in the preheated oven for 12-15 minutes, or until the eggs are set to your desired level of doneness.
6. Remove from the oven, let cool slightly, and carefully remove the egg cups from the muffin tin.
7. Serve warm and enjoy!

Ham and Swiss Breakfast Casserole:

Ingredients:

- 8 eggs
- 1 cup diced ham
- 1/2 cup shredded Swiss cheese
- 1/2 cup diced bell peppers
- 1/4 cup chopped green onions
- 1/4 cup milk or cream
- Salt and pepper to taste

Instructions:

1. Preheat the oven to 375ºF (190ºC) and lightly grease a baking dish with cooking spray.
2. In a mixing bowl, beat the eggs and whisk in the milk or cream until well combined.
3. Spread diced ham, shredded Swiss cheese, diced bell peppers, and chopped green onions evenly in the prepared baking dish.
4. Pour the egg mixture over the ingredients in the baking dish.
5. Season with salt and pepper to taste.
6. Bake in the preheated oven for 25-30 minutes, or until the eggs are set and the top is golden brown.
7. Remove from the oven, let cool slightly, and slice into squares.
8. Serve warm and enjoy!

Caprese Egg Bake:

Ingredients:

- 6 eggs
- 1 cup cherry tomatoes, halved
- 1/2 cup fresh mozzarella cheese, diced

- 2 tablespoons chopped fresh basil
- Salt and pepper to taste
- Cooking spray

Instructions:

1. Preheat the oven to 375°F (190°C) and lightly grease a baking dish with cooking spray.
2. In a mixing bowl, beat the eggs and season with salt and pepper.
3. Spread cherry tomatoes and fresh mozzarella cheese evenly in the prepared baking dish.
4. Pour the beaten eggs over the tomatoes and cheese.
5. Sprinkle chopped fresh basil over the eggs.
6. Bake in the preheated oven for 20-25 minutes, or until the eggs are set and the top is golden brown.
7. Remove from the oven, let cool slightly, and slice into squares.
8. Serve warm and enjoy!

Southwest Egg Burritos:

Ingredients:

- 4 large eggs
- 1/2 cup black beans, drained and rinsed
- 1/4 cup diced red bell pepper
- 1/4 cup diced green bell pepper
- 1/4 cup diced onion
- 1/4 cup shredded cheddar cheese
- 2 tablespoons chopped fresh cilantro
- Salt and pepper to taste
- 4 whole wheat tortillas

Instructions:

1. In a bowl, beat the eggs and season with salt and pepper.
2. Heat a skillet over medium heat and add the beaten eggs.
3. Cook, stirring occasionally, until the eggs are scrambled and cooked through.
4. Add black beans, diced red bell pepper, diced green bell pepper, and diced onion to the skillet.
5. Cook, stirring occasionally, until the vegetables are tender, about 3-4 minutes.
6. Sprinkle shredded cheddar cheese over the egg and vegetable mixture.
7. Spoon the egg and vegetable mixture onto whole wheat tortillas.
8. Roll up the tortillas to form burritos.
9. Serve hot, garnished with chopped fresh cilantro, if desired.

Veggie Breakfast Casserole:

Ingredients:

- 8 eggs
- 1 cup diced bell peppers (any color)
- 1 cup diced onions
- 1 cup diced zucchini
- 1 cup diced tomatoes
- 1 cup shredded cheddar cheese
- 1/2 cup milk or cream
- Salt and pepper to taste

Instructions:

1. Preheat the oven to 375°F (190°C) and lightly grease a baking dish with cooking spray.
2. In a mixing bowl, beat the eggs and whisk in the milk or cream until well combined.
3. Spread diced bell peppers, onions, zucchini, and tomatoes evenly in the prepared baking dish.
4. Pour the egg mixture over the vegetables in the baking dish.
5. Sprinkle shredded cheddar cheese over the egg and vegetable mixture.
6. Season with salt and pepper to taste.
7. Bake in the preheated oven for 25-30 minutes, or until the eggs are set and the top is golden brown.
8. Remove from the oven, let cool slightly, and slice into squares.
9. Serve warm and enjoy!

Kale and Tomato Egg Cups:

Ingredients:

- 6 eggs
- 1 cup chopped kale
- 1/2 cup diced tomatoes
- 1/4 cup shredded mozzarella cheese
- Salt and pepper to taste
- Cooking spray

Instructions:

1. Preheat the oven to 375°F (190°C) and lightly grease a muffin tin with cooking spray.
2. Crack an egg into each muffin cup.
3. Divide chopped kale and diced tomatoes evenly among the muffin cups.
4. Sprinkle shredded mozzarella cheese over each egg cup.
5. Season each egg cup with salt and pepper to taste.

6. Bake in the preheated oven for 12-15 minutes, or until the eggs are set to your desired level of doneness.
7. Remove from the oven, let cool slightly, and carefully remove the egg cups from the muffin tin.
8. Serve warm and enjoy!

Bacon and Spinach Quiche:

Ingredients:

- 1 pie crust (store-bought or homemade)
- 4 eggs
- 1/2 cup cooked and crumbled bacon
- 1 cup chopped spinach
- 1/2 cup shredded cheddar cheese
- 1/2 cup milk or cream
- Salt and pepper to taste
- Cooking spray

Instructions:

1. Preheat the oven to 375°F (190°C) and place the pie crust in a pie dish, pressing it firmly into the bottom and sides.
2. In a mixing bowl, beat the eggs and whisk in the milk or cream until well combined.
3. Spread cooked and crumbled bacon, chopped spinach, and shredded cheddar cheese evenly in the prepared pie crust.
4. Pour the egg mixture over the ingredients in the pie crust.
5. Season with salt and pepper to taste.
6. Bake in the preheated oven for 35-40 minutes, or until the filling is set and the top is golden brown.
7. Remove from the oven, let cool slightly, and slice into wedges.
8. Serve warm or at room temperature, and enjoy!

Greek Yogurt Egg Salad:

Ingredients:

- 6 hard-boiled eggs, chopped
- 1/2 cup Greek yogurt
- 2 tablespoons chopped fresh dill
- 1 tablespoon Dijon mustard
- 1 tablespoon lemon juice
- Salt and pepper to taste

Instructions:

1. In a mixing bowl, combine chopped hard-boiled eggs, Greek yogurt, chopped fresh dill, Dijon mustard, and lemon juice.

2. Mix until well combined.
3. Season with salt and pepper to taste.
4. Serve as a sandwich filling, on top of greens, or with whole grain crackers.
5. Enjoy chilled or at room temperature!

Avocado Egg Salad Wraps:

Ingredients:

- 6 hard-boiled eggs, chopped
- 1 ripe avocado, mashed
- 2 tablespoons Greek yogurt
- 1 tablespoon lemon juice
- Salt and pepper to taste
- 4 large lettuce leaves
- 4 whole grain wraps or tortillas

Instructions:

1. In a mixing bowl, combine chopped hard-boiled eggs, mashed avocado, Greek yogurt, and lemon juice.
2. Mix until well combined.
3. Season with salt and pepper to taste.
4. Lay out the lettuce leaves on each wrap or tortilla.
5. Spoon the avocado egg salad mixture onto the lettuce leaves.
6. Roll up the wraps tightly.
7. Slice in half, if desired, and serve immediately.

Egg and Veggie Breakfast Burritos:

Ingredients:

- 4 large eggs
- 1/2 cup diced bell peppers (any color)
- 1/2 cup diced onions
- 1/2 cup diced tomatoes
- 1/4 cup shredded cheddar cheese
- 1/4 cup salsa
- 4 whole wheat tortillas

Instructions:

1. In a bowl, beat the eggs and season with salt and pepper.
2. Heat a skillet over medium heat and add the beaten eggs.
3. Cook, stirring occasionally, until the eggs are scrambled and cooked through.
4. Add diced bell peppers, onions, and tomatoes to the skillet.
5. Cook, stirring occasionally, until the vegetables are tender, about 3-4 minutes.

6. Divide the scrambled egg and veggie mixture evenly among the tortillas.
7. Sprinkle shredded cheddar cheese over each tortilla.
8. Spoon salsa over the cheese.
9. Roll up the tortillas tightly.
10. Serve hot, and enjoy!

Mediterranean Veggie Omelet:

Ingredients:

- 4 eggs
- 1/4 cup diced bell peppers (any color)
- 1/4 cup diced red onions
- 1/4 cup diced tomatoes
- 1/4 cup chopped spinach
- 1/4 cup crumbled feta cheese
- Salt and pepper to taste
- 1 tablespoon olive oil

Instructions:

1. In a mixing bowl, beat the eggs and season with salt and pepper.
2. Heat olive oil in a non-stick skillet over medium heat.
3. Add diced bell peppers and onions to the skillet and sauté until softened, about 2-3 minutes.
4. Add diced tomatoes and chopped spinach to the skillet and cook until spinach is wilted, about 1-2 minutes.
5. Pour the beaten eggs into the skillet over the veggies.
6. Cook, lifting the edges occasionally, until the eggs are mostly set.
7. Sprinkle crumbled feta cheese over one half of the omelet.
8. Carefully fold the other half of the omelet over the filling.
9. Cook for another 1-2 minutes until the cheese is melted and the omelet is cooked through.
10. Slide onto a plate, cut in half, and serve hot.

Spinach and Tomato Egg Cups:

Ingredients:

- 6 eggs
- 1 cup chopped spinach
- 1/2 cup diced tomatoes
- 1/4 cup shredded mozzarella cheese
- Salt and pepper to taste
- Cooking spray

Instructions:

1. Preheat the oven to 375°F (190°C) and lightly grease a muffin tin with cooking spray.
2. Crack an egg into each muffin cup.
3. Divide chopped spinach and diced tomatoes evenly among the muffin cups.
4. Sprinkle shredded mozzarella cheese over each egg cup.
5. Season each egg cup with salt and pepper to taste.
6. Bake in the preheated oven for 12-15 minutes, or until the eggs are set to your desired level of doneness.
7. Remove from the oven, let cool slightly, and carefully remove the egg cups from the muffin tin.
8. Serve warm and enjoy!

Broccoli Cheddar Egg Muffins:

Ingredients:

- 6 eggs
- 1 cup chopped broccoli florets
- 1/2 cup shredded cheddar cheese
- Salt and pepper to taste
- Cooking spray

Instructions:

1. Preheat the oven to 375°F (190°C) and lightly grease a muffin tin with cooking spray.
2. In a mixing bowl, beat the eggs and season with salt and pepper.
3. Divide chopped broccoli florets evenly among the muffin cups.
4. Pour the beaten eggs over the broccoli in the muffin cups.
5. Sprinkle shredded cheddar cheese over each egg cup.
6. Bake in the preheated oven for 12-15 minutes, or until the eggs are set to your desired level of doneness.
7. Remove from the oven, let cool slightly, and carefully remove the egg cups from the muffin tin.
8. Serve warm and enjoy!

Chapter 3

Midday Bliss: Lunchtime Delights

As the midday sun reaches its zenith, it's time to refuel your body and invigorate your senses with a spread of satisfying lunchtime delights. In this chapter, we'll explore a variety of flavorful dishes designed to tantalize your taste buds and nourish your body, all while keeping acid reflux at bay.

From light and refreshing salads bursting with vibrant colors and textures to comforting soups that warm the soul, our lunchtime repertoire offers something for every palate and preference. Whether you're seeking a quick and easy option for a busy workday or craving a leisurely meal to savor on a lazy afternoon, we've got you covered with recipes that strike the perfect balance between flavor and digestive comfort.

Say goodbye to the monotony of uninspired lunches and embrace a world of culinary possibilities that prioritize both taste and well-being. With our carefully curated selection of lunchtime favorites, you'll never have to sacrifice flavor for digestive peace again.

Indulge in the creamy richness of a roasted vegetable quinoa salad, where tender grains mingle with charred veggies and tangy vinaigrette for a satisfying midday pick-me-up. Or, opt for a hearty grain bowl brimming with wholesome ingredients like avocado, chickpeas, and roasted sweet potatoes, drizzled with a zesty tahini dressing that adds a burst of flavor with every bite. For those craving a taste of the Mediterranean, our Greek-inspired stuffed peppers are sure to delight, filled with a savory mixture of quinoa, spinach, feta cheese, and aromatic herbs. Or, transport your taste buds to the bustling streets of Mexico with our vibrant taco salad bowl, featuring seasoned black beans, crisp lettuce, juicy tomatoes, and creamy avocado, all crowned with a dollop of tangy salsa and a sprinkle of crunchy tortilla strips.

No lunch spread would be complete without a touch of indulgence, and our selection of lunchtime delights includes plenty of options to satisfy your cravings without compromising your digestive health. Treat yourself to a comforting bowl of creamy tomato basil soup, accompanied by a slice of crusty whole grain bread for dipping. Or, whip up a batch of savory mushroom and thyme risotto, where each spoonful is a symphony of earthy flavors and creamy textures that soothe the soul.

Whatever your midday craving may be, our collection of lunchtime delights promises to satisfy your hunger and leave you feeling energized and content. So go ahead, embrace the joy of flavorful, reflux-friendly meals that nourish your body and nurture your well-being, one bite at a time.

Salad

Mixed Green Salad with Grilled Chicken:

Ingredients:

- Mixed greens
- Cherry tomatoes
- Cucumber
- Grilled chicken breast
- Olive oil
- Lemon juice
- Honey
- Salt and pepper

Instructions:

1. Wash and dry the mixed greens, cherry tomatoes, and cucumber. Slice the cherry tomatoes and cucumber.
2. Season the grilled chicken breast with salt and pepper, then grill until cooked through. Slice the chicken into strips.
3. In a small bowl, whisk together olive oil, lemon juice, and honey to make the dressing.
4. In a large bowl, toss the mixed greens, cherry tomatoes, and cucumber with the dressing until evenly coated.
5. Divide the salad among serving plates and top with the sliced grilled chicken breast. Serve immediately.

Spinach and Strawberry Salad:

Ingredients:

- Fresh spinach leaves
- Strawberries
- Goat cheese
- Almonds
- Balsamic vinegar
- Olive oil
- Dijon mustard
- Salt and pepper

Instructions:

1. Wash and dry the spinach leaves and strawberries. Remove the stems from the strawberries and slice them.
2. Crumble the goat cheese and chop the almonds.
3. In a small bowl, whisk together balsamic vinegar, olive oil, Dijon mustard, salt, and pepper to make the dressing.

4. In a large bowl, combine the spinach leaves, sliced strawberries, crumbled goat cheese, and chopped almonds.
5. Drizzle the dressing over the salad and toss until evenly coated. Serve immediately.

Greek Salad:

Ingredients:

- Romaine lettuce
- Cucumbers
- Cherry tomatoes
- Red onion
- Kalamata olives
- Feta cheese
- Olive oil
- Red wine vinegar
- Dried oregano
- Salt and pepper

Instructions:

1. Wash and chop the romaine lettuce, cucumbers, cherry tomatoes, and red onion.
2. Pit the Kalamata olives if necessary and slice them.
3. Crumble the feta cheese.
4. In a small bowl, whisk together olive oil, red wine vinegar, dried oregano, salt, and pepper to make the dressing.
5. In a large bowl, combine the chopped romaine lettuce, cucumbers, cherry tomatoes, red onion, Kalamata olives, and crumbled feta cheese.
6. Drizzle the dressing over the salad and toss until evenly coated. Serve immediately.

Caprese Salad:

Ingredients:

- Ripe tomatoes
- Fresh mozzarella cheese
- Fresh basil leaves
- Balsamic glaze
- Salt and pepper

Instructions:

1. Wash and slice the tomatoes and fresh mozzarella cheese into thick slices.
2. Arrange the tomato and mozzarella slices alternately on a serving platter.
3. Place fresh basil leaves between the tomato and mozzarella slices.
4. Drizzle balsamic glaze over the salad.

5. Sprinkle it with salt and pepper to taste. Serve immediately.

Mediterranean Chickpea Salad:

Ingredients:

- Chickpeas (cooked or canned)
- Cucumbers
- Cherry tomatoes
- Red onion
- Kalamata olives
- Feta cheese
- Olive oil
- Lemon juice
- Garlic (minced)
- Fresh oregano (chopped)
- Salt and pepper

Instructions:

1. Rinse and drain the chickpeas if using canned food.
2. Dice the cucumbers, halve the cherry tomatoes, thinly slice the red onion, and pit the Kalamata olives if necessary.
3. Crumble the feta cheese.
4. In a small bowl, whisk together olive oil, lemon juice, minced garlic, chopped fresh oregano, salt, and pepper to make the dressing.
5. In a large bowl, combine the chickpeas, diced cucumbers, halved cherry tomatoes, sliced red onion, Kalamata olives, and crumbled feta cheese.
6. Pour the dressing over the salad and toss until well coated. Serve immediately.

Arugula and Pear Salad:

Ingredients:

- Arugula
- Pears
- Walnuts
- Parmesan cheese
- Olive oil
- Lemon juice
- Honey
- Dijon mustard
- Salt and pepper

Instructions:

1. Wash and dry the arugula leaves.
2. Core and thinly slice the pears.
3. Toast the walnuts in a dry skillet over medium heat until fragrant, then chop them.
4. Shave the Parmesan cheese using a vegetable peeler.

5. In a small bowl, whisk together olive oil, lemon juice, honey, Dijon mustard, salt, and pepper to make the dressing.
6. In a large bowl, combine the arugula, sliced pears, chopped walnuts, and shaved Parmesan cheese.
7. Drizzle the dressing over the salad and toss until evenly coated. Serve immediately.

Watermelon and Feta Salad:

Ingredients:

- Watermelon
- Feta cheese
- Fresh mint leaves
- Red onion
- Balsamic glaze
- Salt and pepper

Instructions:

1. Cut the watermelon into bite-sized cubes or use a melon baller to create small spheres.
2. Crumble the feta cheese.
3. Thinly slice the red onion.
4. Wash and chop the fresh mint leaves.
5. In a large bowl, combine the watermelon cubes, crumbled feta cheese, sliced red onion, and chopped fresh mint leaves.
6. Drizzle with balsamic glaze and season with salt and pepper to taste.
7. Gently toss the salad until all ingredients are evenly distributed. Serve immediately.

Asian-Inspired Cabbage Salad:

Ingredients:

- Napa cabbage
- Carrots
- Snow peas
- Cilantro
- Sesame seeds (toasted)
- Rice vinegar
- Soy sauce
- Sesame oil
- Honey
- Garlic (minced)
- Ginger (minced)

Instructions:

1. Shred the Napa cabbage and julienne the carrots.
2. Remove the strings from the snow peas and slice them thinly.
3. Wash and chop the cilantro.
4. In a small bowl, whisk together rice vinegar, soy sauce, sesame

oil, honey, minced garlic, and minced ginger to make the dressing.

5. In a large bowl, combine the shredded Napa cabbage, julienned carrots, sliced snow peas, chopped cilantro, and toasted sesame seeds.

6. Pour the dressing over the salad and toss until all ingredients are well coated. Serve immediately.

Mango and Avocado Salad:

Ingredients:

- Mixed greens
- Mango
- Avocado
- Coconut flakes (toasted)
- Macadamia nuts
- Lime
- Ginger (freshly grated)
- Olive oil
- Honey
- Salt and pepper

Instructions:

1. Wash and dry the mixed greens.
2. Peel and dice the mango and avocado.

3. Toast the coconut flakes in a dry skillet over medium heat until golden brown.

4. Chop the macadamia nuts.

5. In a small bowl, whisk together the juice of a lime, freshly grated ginger, olive oil, honey, salt, and pepper to make the dressing.

6. In a large bowl, combine the mixed greens, diced mango, diced avocado, toasted coconut flakes, and chopped macadamia nuts.

7. Drizzle the dressing over the salad and toss gently to coat all ingredients. Serve immediately.

Panzanella Salad:

Ingredients:

- Stale bread (preferably Italian or sourdough)
- Tomatoes
- Cucumber
- Red onion
- Basil leaves
- Balsamic vinegar
- Olive oil
- Garlic (minced)
- Dijon mustard
- Salt and pepper

Instructions:

1. Tear the stale bread into bite-sized pieces and place them in a large bowl.
2. Dice the tomatoes and cucumber.
3. Thinly slice the red onion.
4. Wash and tear the basil leaves.
5. In a small bowl, whisk together balsamic vinegar, olive oil, minced garlic, Dijon mustard, salt, and pepper to make the dressing.
6. Add the diced tomatoes, diced cucumber, sliced red onion, and torn basil leaves to the bowl with the bread.
7. Drizzle the dressing over the salad and toss gently to combine. Let the salad sit for at least 10 minutes to allow the bread to soak up the flavors. Serve at room temperature.

Cucumber and Dill Salad:

Ingredients:

- English cucumbers
- Red onion
- Fresh dill
- Feta cheese
- Lemon
- Olive oil
- Garlic (minced)
- Salt and pepper

Instructions:

1. Thinly slice the English cucumbers and red onion.
2. Chop the fresh dill.
3. Crumble the feta cheese.
4. In a small bowl, whisk together the juice of a lemon, olive oil, minced garlic, salt, and pepper to make the dressing.
5. In a large bowl, combine the sliced cucumbers, sliced red onion, chopped dill, and crumbled feta cheese.
6. Drizzle the dressing over the salad and toss gently to coat. Serve immediately.

Black Bean and Corn Salad:

Ingredients:

- Black beans (cooked or canned)
- Corn kernels (fresh or frozen)
- Red bell pepper
- Red onion
- Cilantro
- Lime
- Olive oil

- Cumin
- Salt and pepper

Instructions:

1. Rinse and drain the black beans if using canned.
2. If using fresh corn, cook the corn kernels in boiling water for 3-5 minutes, then drain. If using frozen, thaw the corn kernels.
3. Dice the red bell pepper and red onion.
4. Chop the cilantro.
5. In a small bowl, whisk together the juice of a lime, olive oil, ground cumin, salt, and pepper to make the dressing.
6. In a large bowl, combine the black beans, corn kernels, diced red bell pepper, diced red onion, and chopped cilantro.
7. Pour the dressing over the salad and toss gently to coat. Serve chilled or at room temperature.

Mango and Avocado Salad:

Ingredients:

- Arugula
- Mango
- Avocado
- Toasted coconut flakes
- Chopped macadamia nuts
- Lime
- Ginger (freshly grated)
- Olive oil
- Honey
- Salt and pepper

Instructions:

1. Wash and dry the arugula.
2. Peel and dice the mango and avocado.
3. Toast the coconut flakes in a dry skillet over medium heat until golden brown.
4. In a small bowl, whisk together the juice of a lime, freshly grated ginger, olive oil, honey, salt, and pepper to make the dressing.
5. In a large bowl, combine the arugula, diced mango, diced avocado, toasted coconut flakes, and chopped macadamia nuts.
6. Drizzle the dressing over the salad and toss gently to coat. Serve immediately.

Panzanella Salad:

Ingredients:

- Stale bread (preferably Italian or sourdough)

- Tomatoes
- Cucumber
- Red onion
- Basil leaves
- Balsamic vinegar
- Olive oil
- Garlic (minced)
- Salt and pepper

Instructions:

1. Tear the stale bread into bite-sized pieces and place them in a large bowl.
2. Dice the tomatoes and cucumber.
3. Thinly slice the red onion.
4. Wash and tear the basil leaves.
5. In a small bowl, whisk together balsamic vinegar, olive oil, minced garlic, salt, and pepper to make the dressing.
6. Add the diced tomatoes, diced cucumber, sliced red onion, and torn basil leaves to the bowl with the bread.
7. Drizzle the dressing over the salad and toss gently to combine. Let the salad sit for at least 10 minutes to allow the bread to soak up the flavors. Serve at room temperature.

Fruit and Nut Salad:

Ingredients:

- Mixed greens
- Apples
- Grapes
- Dried cranberries
- Toasted almonds
- Honey
- Poppy seeds
- Olive oil
- Lemon juice
- Dijon mustard
- Salt and pepper

Instructions:

1. Wash and dry the mixed greens.
2. Core and dice the apples.
3. Wash and halve the grapes.
4. In a small bowl, whisk together honey, poppy seeds, olive oil, lemon juice, Dijon mustard, salt, and pepper to make the dressing.
5. In a large bowl, combine the mixed greens, diced apples, halved grapes, dried cranberries, and toasted almonds.
6. Drizzle the dressing over the salad and toss gently to coat. Serve immediately.

Chickpea and Roasted Vegetable Salad:

Ingredients:

- Roasted vegetables (such as bell peppers, zucchini, and eggplant)
- Cooked chickpeas
- Chopped fresh herbs (such as parsley and thyme)
- Crumbled feta cheese
- Lemon
- Tahini
- Olive oil
- Garlic (minced)
- Salt and pepper

Instructions:

1. Prepare the roasted vegetables and cooked chickpeas if not already done.
2. Chop the fresh herbs.
3. Crumble the feta cheese.
4. In a small bowl, whisk together the juice of a lemon, tahini, olive oil, minced garlic, salt, and pepper to make the dressing.
5. In a large bowl, combine the roasted vegetables, cooked chickpeas, chopped fresh herbs, and crumbled feta cheese.
6. Drizzle the dressing over the salad and toss gently to coat. Serve immediately.

Shaved Brussels Sprouts Salad:

Ingredients:

- Brussels sprouts
- Apples
- Dried cranberries
- Chopped pecans
- Crumbled blue cheese
- Maple syrup
- Dijon mustard
- Apple cider vinegar
- Olive oil
- Salt and pepper

Instructions:

1. Shave the Brussels sprouts thinly using a sharp knife or mandolin slicer.
2. Core and thinly slice the apples.
3. In a small bowl, whisk together maple syrup, Dijon mustard, apple cider vinegar, olive oil, salt, and pepper to make the dressing.
4. In a large bowl, combine the shaved Brussels sprouts, sliced apples, dried cranberries,

chopped pecans, and crumbled blue cheese.

5. Drizzle the dressing over the salad and toss gently to coat. Serve immediately.

Taco Salad:

Ingredients:

- Mixed greens
- Cooked ground turkey
- Black beans (cooked or canned)
- Diced tomatoes
- Shredded cheddar cheese
- Crushed tortilla chips
- Avocado
- Greek yogurt
- Lime juice
- Cilantro
- Garlic powder
- Salt and pepper

Instructions:

1. Wash and dry the mixed greens.
2. Cook the ground turkey in a skillet over medium heat until browned and cooked through. Season with salt, pepper, and garlic powder.
3. Rinse and drain the black beans if using canned.
4. Dice the tomatoes and avocado.
5. In a small bowl, mash the avocado with Greek yogurt, lime juice, chopped cilantro, garlic powder, salt, and pepper to make the creamy avocado dressing.
6. In a large bowl, combine the mixed greens, cooked ground turkey, black beans, diced tomatoes, shredded cheddar cheese, and crushed tortilla chips.
7. Drizzle the creamy avocado dressing over the salad and toss gently to coat. Serve immediately.

Israeli Couscous Salad:

Ingredients:

- Israeli couscous (cooked)
- Cucumbers
- Cherry tomatoes
- Kalamata olives
- Feta cheese
- Parsley
- Olive oil
- Lemon juice
- Garlic (minced)
- Salt and pepper

Instructions:

1. Cook the Israeli couscous according to package instructions and let it cool.
2. Dice the cucumbers and halve the cherry tomatoes.
3. Pit the Kalamata olives if necessary.
4. Crumble the feta cheese.
5. In a small bowl, whisk together olive oil, lemon juice, minced garlic, salt, and pepper to make the lemon-herb vinaigrette.
6. In a large bowl, combine the cooked Israeli couscous, diced cucumbers, halved cherry tomatoes, Kalamata olives, crumbled feta cheese, and chopped parsley.
7. Drizzle the lemon-herb vinaigrette over the salad and toss gently to coat. Serve chilled or at room temperature.

Waldorf Salad:

Ingredients:

- Apples
- Celery
- Grapes
- Walnuts
- Greek yogurt
- Honey
- Mixed greens

Instructions:

1. Core and dice the apples.
2. Slice the celery and halve the grapes.
3. Toast the walnuts in a dry skillet over medium heat until fragrant.
4. In a small bowl, whisk together Greek yogurt and honey to taste.
5. In a large bowl, combine the diced apples, sliced celery, halved grapes, and toasted walnuts.
6. Add the Greek yogurt dressing to the salad and toss gently to coat.
7. Serve the Waldorf salad on a bed of mixed greens.

Asian Pear Salad:

Ingredients:

- Asian pears
- Mixed greens
- Radishes
- Almonds
- Goat cheese
- Soy sauce
- Rice vinegar
- Sesame oil

- Honey
- Ginger (minced)

Instructions:

1. Thinly slice the Asian pears.
2. Wash and dry the mixed greens and radishes.
3. Toast the almonds in a dry skillet over medium heat until golden brown.
4. In a small bowl, whisk together soy sauce, rice vinegar, sesame oil, honey, and minced ginger to make the ginger-soy vinaigrette.
5. In a large bowl, combine the sliced Asian pears, mixed greens, thinly sliced radishes, toasted almonds, and crumbled goat cheese.
6. Drizzle the ginger-soy vinaigrette over the salad and toss gently to coat. Serve immediately.

Mediterranean Orzo Salad:

Ingredients:

- Orzo (cooked)
- Cucumbers
- Cherry tomatoes
- Kalamata olives
- Feta cheese
- Parsley
- Olive oil
- Lemon juice
- Garlic (minced)
- Salt and pepper

Instructions:

1. Cook the orzo according to package instructions and let it cool.
2. Dice the cucumbers and halve the cherry tomatoes.
3. Pit the Kalamata olives if necessary.
4. Crumble the feta cheese.
5. In a small bowl, whisk together olive oil, lemon juice, minced garlic, salt, and pepper to make the lemon-garlic vinaigrette.
6. In a large bowl, combine the cooked orzo, diced cucumbers, halved cherry tomatoes, Kalamata olives, crumbled feta cheese, and chopped parsley.
7. Drizzle the lemon-garlic vinaigrette over the salad and toss gently to coat. Serve chilled or at room temperature.

Soups

Creamy Butternut Squash Soup:

Ingredients:

- 1 medium butternut squash, peeled, seeded, and cubed
- 1 onion, chopped
- 2 cloves garlic, minced
- 4 cups vegetable broth
- 1 teaspoon ground cinnamon
- 1/2 teaspoon ground nutmeg
- Salt and pepper to taste
- Olive oil for sautéing
- Optional: 1/2 cup coconut milk for extra creaminess

Instructions:

1. In a large pot, heat olive oil over medium heat. Add chopped onion and minced garlic, and sauté until softened.
2. Add cubed butternut squash to the pot and cook for 5 minutes, stirring occasionally.
3. Pour in vegetable broth and bring to a boil. Reduce heat to low, cover, and simmer for 20–25 minutes, or until squash is tender.
4. Use an immersion blender to puree the soup until smooth. Alternatively, transfer the soup to add batches to a blender and blend until smooth.
5. Stir in ground cinnamon, ground nutmeg, salt, and pepper to taste. If desired, add coconut milk for extra creaminess.
6. Simmer for an additional 5 minutes to allow flavors to meld. Adjust seasoning if needed.
7. Serve hot, garnished with a drizzle of coconut milk or a sprinkle of fresh herbs, if desired.

Cooking Time: 35-40 minutes
Serving Size: 4-6 servings

Pro Tips:

- For a time-saving option, use pre-cut butternut squash from the grocery store.
- Adjust the consistency of the soup by adding more or less vegetable broth according to your preference.

Ginger Carrot Soup:

Ingredients:

- 1 lb. carrots, peeled and chopped
- 1 onion, chopped
- 2 cloves garlic, minced
- 1 tablespoon fresh ginger, grated
- 4 cups vegetable broth
- 1 tablespoon olive oil
- Salt and pepper to taste
- Fresh cilantro for garnish (optional)

Instructions:

1. In a large pot, heat olive oil over medium heat. Add chopped onion and cook until translucent.
2. Add minced garlic and grated ginger to the pot, and cook for an additional 2 minutes.
3. Add chopped carrots and vegetable broth to the pot. Bring to a boil, then reduce heat to low, cover, and simmer for 20-25 minutes, or until carrots are tender.
4. Use an immersion blender to puree the soup until smooth. Alternatively, transfer the soup in batches to a blender and blend until smooth.
5. Season with salt and pepper, to taste. Adjust seasoning if needed.
6. Serve hot, garnished with fresh cilantro if desired.

Cooking Time: 30-35 minutes
Serving Size: 4-6 servings

Pro Tips:

- For added depth of flavor, roast the carrots in the oven before adding them to the soup.
- Garnish with a dollop of Greek yogurt or a swirl of coconut cream for extra creaminess.

Turmeric Lentil Soup:

Ingredients:

- 1 cup dried red lentils, rinsed
- 1 onion, chopped
- 2 cloves garlic, minced
- 1 tablespoon fresh ginger, grated
- 1 teaspoon ground turmeric
- 4 cups vegetable broth
- 1 cup canned diced tomatoes
- 1 tablespoon olive oil
- Salt and pepper to taste
- Fresh cilantro for garnish (optional)

Instructions:

1. In a large pot, heat olive oil over medium heat. Add chopped onion and cook until translucent.
2. Add minced garlic and grated ginger to the pot, and cook for an additional 2 minutes.
3. Stir in ground turmeric and cook for 1 minute, until fragrant.
4. Add rinsed red lentils, vegetable broth, and diced tomatoes to the pot. Bring to a boil, then reduce heat to low, cover, and simmer for 20-25 minutes, or until lentils are tender.
5. Use an immersion blender to partially puree the soup, leaving some lentils whole for texture. Alternatively, transfer a portion of the soup to a blender and blend until smooth, then return to the pot.
6. Season with salt and pepper, to taste. Adjust seasoning if needed.
7. Serve hot, garnished with fresh cilantro if desired.

Cooking Time: 30-35 minutes
Serving Size: 4-6 servings

Pro Tips:

- For added protein, stir in a handful of cooked quinoas or diced cooked chicken before serving.
- Turmeric can stain surfaces easily, so be cautious when handling it to avoid stains.

Coconut Cauliflower Soup:

Ingredients:

- 1 medium cauliflower, chopped into florets
- 1 onion, chopped
- 2 cloves garlic, minced
- 1 can (14 oz) coconut milk
- 4 cups vegetable broth
- 1 tablespoon curry powder
- 1 tablespoon olive oil
- Salt and pepper to taste
- Fresh cilantro for garnish (optional)

Instructions:

1. In a large pot, heat olive oil over medium heat. Add the chopped onion and cook until translucent.
2. Add minced garlic to the pot, and cook for an additional 2 minutes.
3. Add chopped cauliflower, curry powder, coconut milk, and vegetable broth to the pot. Bring

to a boil, then reduce heat to low, cover, and simmer for 20-25 minutes, or until cauliflower is tender.

4. Use an immersion blender to puree the soup until smooth. Alternatively, transfer the soup in batches to a blender and blend until smooth.
5. Season with salt and pepper, to taste. Adjust seasoning if needed.
6. Serve hot, garnished with fresh cilantro if desired.

Cooking Time: 30-35 minutes
Serving Size: 4-6 servings

Pro Tips:

- For extra richness, use full-fat coconut milk.
- Feel free to add a dash of cayenne pepper for a spicy kick.

Spinach and Potato Soup:

Ingredients:

- 4 medium potatoes, peeled and diced
- 1 onion, chopped
- 2 cloves garlic, minced
- 4 cups vegetable broth
- 4 cups fresh spinach leaves
- 1 tablespoon olive oil
- Salt and pepper to taste
- Fresh parsley for garnish (optional)

Instructions:

1. In a large pot, heat olive oil over medium heat. Add chopped onion and cook until translucent.
2. Add minced garlic to the pot, and cook for an additional 2 minutes.
3. Add diced potatoes and vegetable broth to the pot. Bring to a boil, then reduce heat to low, cover, and simmer for 15-20 minutes, or until potatoes are tender.
4. Stir in fresh spinach leaves and cook for an additional 2-3 minutes, until wilted.
5. Use an immersion blender to partially puree the soup, leaving some chunks of potato for texture. Alternatively, transfer a portion of the soup to a blender and blend until smooth, then return it to the pot.
6. Season with salt and pepper, to taste. Adjust seasoning if needed.
7. Serve hot, garnished with fresh parsley if desired.

Cooking Time: 25-30 minutes
Serving Size: 4-6 servings

Pro Tips:

- For added creaminess, stir in a splash of coconut milk or Greek yogurt before serving.
- Feel free to add other vegetables, such as carrots or celery, for extra flavor and nutrition.

Creamy Mushroom Soup:

Ingredients:

- 1 lb. mushrooms, sliced
- 1 onion, chopped
- 2 cloves garlic, minced
- 4 cups vegetable broth
- 1 cup unsweetened almond milk
- 2 tablespoons olive oil
- 2 tablespoons all-purpose flour (optional, for thickening)
- Salt and pepper to taste
- Fresh thyme for garnish (optional)

Instructions:

1. In a large pot, heat olive oil over medium heat. Add chopped onion and cook until translucent.
2. Add sliced mushrooms to the pot and cook until browned and tender.
3. Add minced garlic to the pot and cook for an additional 2 minutes.
4. If using, sprinkle all-purpose flour over the mushrooms and stir to coat.
5. Gradually pour in vegetable broth and almond milk, stirring constantly to prevent lumps from forming.
6. Bring the soup to a simmer and cook for 10-15 minutes, or until slightly thickened.
7. Season with salt and pepper, to taste. Adjust seasoning if needed.
8. Serve hot, garnished with fresh thyme if desired.

Cooking Time: 25-30 minutes
Serving Size: 4-6 servings

Pro Tips:

- For extra richness, substitute half of the almond milk with coconut milk or cream.

- For a smoother texture, blend a portion of the soup until smooth before serving.

Zucchini Basil Soup:

Ingredients:

- 4 medium zucchinis, chopped
- 1 onion, chopped
- 2 cloves garlic, minced
- 4 cups vegetable broth
- 1 cup fresh basil leaves
- 1 tablespoon olive oil
- Salt and pepper to taste
- Fresh basil leaves for garnish (optional)

Instructions:

1. In a large pot, heat olive oil over medium heat. Add chopped onion and cook until translucent.
2. Add minced garlic to the pot and cook for an additional 2 minutes.
3. Add chopped zucchinis to the pot and cook until softened, about 5-7 minutes.
4. Pour in vegetable broth and bring to a boil. Reduce heat to low, cover, and simmer for 15-20 minutes, or until zucchinis are tender.
5. Stir in fresh basil leaves and cook for an additional 2-3 minutes, until wilted.
6. Use an immersion blender to puree the soup until smooth. Alternatively, transfer the soup in batches to a blender and blend until smooth.
7. Season with salt and pepper, to taste. Adjust seasoning if needed.
8. Serve hot, garnished with fresh basil leaves if desired.

Cooking Time: 25-30 minutes
Serving Size: 4-6 servings

Pro Tips:

- For added creaminess, stir in a splash of coconut milk or Greek yogurt before serving.
- Garnish with a drizzle of extra virgin olive oil or a sprinkle of grated Parmesan cheese for extra flavor.

Roasted Red Pepper Soup:

Ingredients:

- 4 large red bell peppers, halved and seeded
- 1 onion, chopped

- 2 cloves garlic, minced
- 4 cups low-sodium chicken or vegetable broth
- 1 teaspoon smoked paprika
- Salt and pepper, to taste
- Olive oil, for roasting

Instructions:

1. Preheat the oven to 400°F (200°C). Place the red bell pepper halves on a baking sheet, cut side down. Drizzle with olive oil, and season with salt and pepper.
2. Roast the peppers in the preheated oven for 25-30 minutes, or until the skins are blistered and charred.
3. Remove the peppers from the oven and let them cool slightly. Peel off the charred skins and discard.
4. In a large pot, heat some olive oil over medium heat. Add the chopped onion and garlic, and sauté until softened, about 5 minutes.
5. Add the roasted red peppers, chicken or vegetable broth, and smoked paprika to the pot. Bring to a simmer and cook for 10-15 minutes.
6. Use an immersion blender to puree the soup until smooth. Alternatively, transfer the soup to a blender and blend until smooth.
7. Season the soup with salt and pepper to taste. Serve hot, garnished with a drizzle of olive oil or a dollop of Greek yogurt, if desired.

Cooking Time: 45 minutes
Serving Size: 4 servings

Pro Tip: For extra flavor, you can add a pinch of red pepper flakes or a splash of balsamic vinegar to the soup before serving.

Lemon Chicken Orzo Soup:

Ingredients:

- 1 tablespoon olive oil
- 1 onion, diced
- 2 carrots, diced
- 2 celery stalks, diced
- 2 cloves garlic, minced
- 6 cups low-sodium chicken broth
- 1 cup cooked chicken, shredded or diced
- 1/2 cup uncooked orzo pasta
- Juice of 1 lemon
- Salt and pepper, to taste

- Fresh parsley, for garnish

Instructions:

1. In a large pot, heat the olive oil over medium heat. Add the diced onion, carrots, and celery, and sauté until softened, about 5 minutes.
2. Add the minced garlic to the pot and sauté for an additional minute, until fragrant.
3. Pour in the chicken broth and bring the soup to a boil. Reduce the heat to low and simmer for 10 minutes.
4. Add the cooked chicken and orzo pasta to the pot. Continue to simmer for another 10-12 minutes, or until the orzo is tender.
5. Stir in the lemon juice, and season the soup with salt and pepper to taste.
6. Ladle the soup into bowls and garnish with fresh parsley before serving.

Cooking Time: 30 minutes
Serving Size: 4 servings

Pro Tip: For added freshness, you can stir in some chopped spinach or kale during the last few minutes of cooking.

Broccoli Cheddar Soup (low-fat version):

Ingredients:

- 1 tablespoon olive oil
- 1 onion, chopped
- 2 cloves garlic, minced
- 4 cups low-sodium vegetable broth
- 1 large head broccoli, chopped (about 4 cups)
- 1 large potato, peeled and diced
- 1 cup unsweetened almond milk
- 1 cup shredded reduced-fat cheddar cheese
- Salt and pepper, to taste

Instructions:

1. In a large pot, heat the olive oil over medium heat. Add the chopped onion and garlic, and sauté until softened, about 5 minutes.
2. Add the vegetable broth, chopped broccoli, and diced potato to the pot. Bring to a boil, then reduce the heat to low and simmer for 15-20 minutes, or until the vegetables are tender.
3. Use an immersion blender to puree the soup until smooth. Alternatively, transfer the soup to a blender and blend until smooth, then return it to the pot.

4. Stir in the almond milk and shredded cheddar cheese until the cheese is melted and the soup is creamy.

5. Season the soup with salt and pepper to taste. Serve hot.

Cooking Time: 30 minutes
Serving Size: 4 servings

Pro Tip: For extra creaminess, you can add a dollop of Greek yogurt or sour cream to each serving before serving.

Sweet Potato and Kale Soup:

Ingredients:

- 2 tablespoons olive oil
- 1 onion, chopped
- 2 cloves garlic, minced
- 2 large sweet potatoes, peeled and diced
- 4 cups low-sodium vegetable broth
- 2 cups chopped kale
- 1 teaspoon ground cumin
- 1/2 teaspoon ground cinnamon
- Salt and pepper, to taste

Instructions:

1. In a large pot, heat the olive oil over medium heat. Add the chopped onion and garlic, and sauté until softened, about 5 minutes.

2. Add the diced sweet potatoes to the pot and sauté for another 5 minutes.

3. Pour in the vegetable broth and bring the soup to a boil. Reduce the heat to low and simmer for 15-20 minutes, or until the sweet potatoes are tender.

4. Stir in the chopped kale, ground cumin, and ground cinnamon. Simmer for an additional 5 minutes, until the kale is wilted.

5. Use an immersion blender to partially puree the soup, leaving some chunks of sweet potato for texture.

6. Season the soup with salt and pepper to taste. Serve hot.

Cooking Time: 30 minutes
Serving Size: 4 servings

Pro Tip: For added protein, you can stir in a can of drained and rinsed white beans or chickpeas during the last few minutes of cooking.

Creamy Tomato Basil Soup (dairy-free):

Ingredients:

- 1 tablespoon olive oil
- 1 onion, chopped
- 2 cloves garlic, minced
- 2 cans (14 ounces each) diced tomatoes
- 2 cups low-sodium vegetable broth
- 1/2 cup unsweetened almond milk
- 1/4 cup chopped fresh basil
- Salt and pepper, to taste;

Instructions:

1. In a large pot, heat the olive oil over medium heat. Add the chopped onion and garlic, and sauté until softened, about 5 minutes.
2. Add the diced tomatoes (with their juices) and vegetable broth to the pot. Bring to a boil, then reduce the heat to low and simmer for 10-15 minutes.
3. Use an immersion blender to puree the soup until smooth. Alternatively, transfer the soup to a blender and blend until smooth, then return it to the pot.
4. Stir in the almond milk and chopped basil until well combined. Simmer for another 5 minutes.
5. Season the soup with salt and pepper to taste. Serve hot.

Cooking Time: 25 minutes
Serving Size: 4 servings

Pro Tip: For a burst of freshness, you can add a squeeze of lemon juice to each bowl before serving.

Chicken and Vegetable Soup:

Ingredients:

- 1 tablespoon olive oil
- 1 onion, chopped
- 2 carrots, diced
- 2 celery stalks, diced
- 2 cloves garlic, minced
- 6 cups low-sodium chicken broth
- 2 cups cooked chicken, shredded or diced
- 1 cup diced tomatoes
- 1 cup chopped spinach
- Salt and pepper, to taste

Instructions:

1. In a large pot, heat the olive oil over medium heat. Add the

chopped onion, carrots, celery, and garlic, and sauté until softened, about 5 minutes.

2. Pour in the chicken broth and bring the soup to a boil. Reduce the heat to low and simmer for 10 minutes.
3. Add the cooked chicken, diced tomatoes, and chopped spinach to the pot. Continue to simmer for another 5 minutes.
4. Season the soup with salt and pepper to taste. Serve hot.

Cooking Time: 20 minutes
Serving Size: 4 servings

Pro Tip: For extra flavor, you can add a sprinkle of dried herbs like thyme or oregano to the soup before serving.

Miso Soup with Tofu and Seaweed:

Ingredients:

- 4 cups water
- 3 tablespoons white miso paste
- 1 cup firm tofu, diced
- 2 green onions, thinly sliced
- 2 sheets nori seaweed, torn into small pieces
- 1 tablespoon soy sauce
- 1 teaspoon sesame oil

Instructions:

1. In a medium pot, bring the water to a simmer over medium heat.
2. In a small bowl, whisk together the miso paste with a few tablespoons of the hot water until smooth.
3. Add the miso mixture to the pot and stir to combine.
4. Add the diced tofu, sliced green onions, torn nori seaweed, soy sauce, and sesame oil to the pot. Simmer for 5-7 minutes, until heated through.
5. Taste the soup and adjust the seasoning with more soy sauce if needed.
6. Serve hot.

Cooking Time: 15 minutes
Serving Size: 4 servings

Pro Tip: Be careful not to boil the miso soup once the miso paste has been added, as boiling can destroy the delicate flavors of the miso.

Acorn Squash Soup with Apple and Sage:

Ingredients:

- 2 acorn squash, halved and seeded
- 2 tablespoons of olive oil
- 1 onion, chopped
- 2 cloves garlic, minced
- 1 apple, peeled, cored, and chopped
- 4 cups low-sodium vegetable broth
- 1 teaspoon dried sage
- Salt and pepper, to taste

Instructions:

1. Preheat the oven to 400°F (200°C). Place the acorn squash halves on a baking sheet, cut side down. Roast in the preheated oven for 30-40 minutes, or until the squash is tender.
2. Remove the squash from the oven and let it cool slightly. Scoop out the flesh and set aside.
3. In a large pot, heat the olive oil over medium heat. Add the chopped onion and garlic, and sauté until softened, about 5 minutes.
4. Add the chopped apple to the pot and sauté for another 2-3 minutes.
5. Add the roasted acorn squash flesh, vegetable broth, and dried sage to the pot. Bring to a boil, then reduce the heat to low and simmer for 10-15 minutes.
6. Use an immersion blender to puree the soup until smooth. Alternatively, transfer the soup to a blender and blend until smooth, then return it to the pot.
7. Season the soup with salt and pepper to taste. Serve hot.

Cooking Time: 50 minutes
Serving Size: 4 servings

Pro Tip: For added richness, you can stir in a splash of coconut milk or heavy cream before serving.

Creamy Asparagus Soup:

Ingredients:

- 1 tablespoon olive oil
- 1 onion, chopped
- 2 cloves garlic, minced
- 1 pound asparagus, tough ends trimmed and chopped

- 4 cups low-sodium vegetable broth
- 1/2 cup unsweetened almond milk
- Salt and pepper, to taste

Instructions:

1. In a large pot, heat the olive oil over medium heat. Add the chopped onion and garlic, and sauté until softened, about 5 minutes.
2. Add the chopped asparagus to the pot and sauté for another 5 minutes.
3. Pour in the vegetable broth and bring the soup to a boil. Reduce the heat to low and simmer for 15-20 minutes, or until the asparagus is tender.
4. Use an immersion blender to puree the soup until smooth. Alternatively, transfer the soup to a blender and blend until smooth, then return it to the pot.
5. Stir in the almond milk until well combined. Simmer for another 5 minutes.
6. Season the soup with salt and pepper to taste. Serve hot.

Cooking Time: 30 minutes
Serving Size: 4 servings

Pro Tip: For added flavor, you can stir in some fresh lemon juice or grated Parmesan cheese before serving.

Thai-Inspired Chicken Soup with Lemongrass:

Ingredients:

- 1 tablespoon olive oil
- 1 onion, chopped
- 2 cloves garlic, minced
- 2 stalks lemongrass, bruised and chopped
- 1 red bell pepper, thinly sliced
- 1 carrot, thinly sliced
- 4 cups low-sodium chicken broth
- 1 can (14 ounces) coconut milk
- 2 cups cooked chicken, shredded or diced
- Juice of 1 lime
- Salt and pepper, to taste
- Fresh cilantro, for garnish

Instructions:

1. In a large pot, heat the olive oil over medium heat. Add the chopped onion and garlic, and sauté until softened, about 5 minutes.

2. Add the chopped lemongrass, sliced red bell pepper, and sliced carrot to the pot. Sauté for another 5 minutes.
3. Pour in the chicken broth and coconut milk, and bring the soup to a boil. Reduce the heat to low and simmer for 10-15 minutes.
4. Add the cooked chicken to the pot and simmer for another 5 minutes.
5. Stir in the lime juice and season the soup with salt and pepper to taste.
6. Ladle the soup into bowls and garnish with fresh cilantro before serving.

Cooking Time: 30 minutes
Serving Size: 4 servings

Pro Tip: For added heat, you can stir in some thinly sliced Thai chili peppers or a drizzle of sriracha sauce before serving.

Quinoa Vegetable Soup:

Ingredients:

- 1 tablespoon olive oil
- 1 onion, chopped
- 2 cloves garlic, minced
- 2 carrots, diced
- 2 celery stalks, diced
- 1 cup diced tomatoes
- 1/2 cup quinoa, rinsed
- 4 cups low-sodium vegetable broth
- 2 cups chopped spinach or kale
- Salt and pepper, to taste
- Fresh parsley, for garnish

Instructions:

1. In a large pot, heat the olive oil over medium heat. Add the chopped onion and garlic, and sauté until softened, about 5 minutes.
2. Add the diced carrots and celery to the pot and sauté for another 5 minutes.
3. Stir in the diced tomatoes, rinsed quinoa, and vegetable broth. Bring the soup to a boil, then reduce the heat to low and simmer for 15-20 minutes, or until the quinoa is cooked and the vegetables are tender.
4. Add the chopped spinach or kale to the pot and simmer for another 5 minutes, until wilted.
5. Season the soup with salt and pepper to taste. Serve hot, garnished with fresh parsley.

Cooking Time: 30 minutes
Serving Size: 4 servings

Pro Tip: For added protein, you can stir in some cooked beans or lentils during the last few minutes of cooking.

Creamy Avocado Soup:

Ingredients:

- 2 ripe avocados, peeled and pitted
- 1 cucumber, peeled and chopped
- 1/4 cup fresh cilantro leaves
- 2 tablespoons lime juice
- 2 cups low-sodium vegetable broth
- Salt and pepper, to taste
- Greek yogurt, for garnish (optional)
- Tortilla strips, for garnish (optional)

Instructions:

1. In a blender, combine the ripe avocados, chopped cucumber, cilantro leaves, lime juice, and vegetable broth. Blend until smooth.
2. Season the soup with salt and pepper to taste. If the soup is too thick, you can add more vegetable broth or water to reach your desired consistency.
3. Transfer the soup to a pot and heat over medium heat until warmed through, stirring occasionally.
4. Ladle the soup into bowls and garnish with a dollop of Greek yogurt and a sprinkle of tortilla strips, if desired.

Cooking Time: 10 minutes
Serving Size: 4 servings

Pro Tip: For added freshness, you can stir in some diced tomatoes or bell peppers before serving.

Lemon Ginger Chicken Soup:

Ingredients:

- 1 tablespoon olive oil
- 1 onion, chopped
- 2 cloves garlic, minced
- 1 tablespoon grated ginger
- 6 cups low-sodium chicken broth
- 2 cups cooked chicken, shredded or diced
- 1 cup chopped carrots
- 1/2 cup orzo pasta
- Juice of 1 lemon

- Salt and pepper, to taste
- Fresh parsley, for garnish

Instructions:

1. In a large pot, heat the olive oil over medium heat. Add the chopped onion and sauté until softened, about 5 minutes.
2. Add the minced garlic and grated ginger to the pot and sauté for another minute, until fragrant.
3. Pour in the chicken broth and bring the soup to a boil. Reduce the heat to low and simmer for 10 minutes.
4. Add the cooked chicken, chopped carrots, and orzo pasta to the pot. Simmer for another 8-10 minutes, or until the orzo is tender.
5. Stir in the lemon juice, and season the soup with salt and pepper to taste.
6. Ladle the soup into bowls and garnish with fresh parsley before serving.

Cooking Time: 25 minutes
Serving Size: 4 servings

Pro Tip: For added flavor, you can stir in some chopped spinach or kale during the last few minutes of cooking.

Pumpkin and Sage Soup:

Ingredients:

- 1 tablespoon olive oil
- 1 onion, chopped
- 2 cloves garlic, minced
- 1 can (15 ounces) pumpkin puree
- 4 cups low-sodium vegetable broth
- 1/2 cup unsweetened coconut milk
- 1 teaspoon dried sage
- Salt and pepper, to taste
- Toasted pumpkin seeds, for garnish (optional)

Instructions:

1. In a large pot, heat the olive oil over medium heat. Add the chopped onion and garlic, and sauté until softened, about 5 minutes.
2. Add the pumpkin puree, vegetable broth, coconut milk, and dried sage to the pot. Bring to a boil, then reduce the heat to low and simmer for 10-15 minutes.
3. Use an immersion blender to puree the soup until smooth.

Alternatively, transfer the soup to a blender and blend until smooth, then return it to the pot.

4. Season the soup with salt and pepper to taste. Serve hot, garnished with toasted pumpkin seeds if desired.

Cooking Time: 20 minutes
Serving Size: 4 servings

Pro Tip: For added richness, you can stir in a dollop of Greek yogurt or sour cream before serving.

Cauliflower and Leek Soup:

Ingredients:

- 1 tablespoon olive oil
- 2 leeks, white and light green parts only, chopped
- 1 head cauliflower, chopped
- 4 cups low-sodium vegetable broth
- 1 cup unsweetened almond milk
- Salt and pepper, to taste
- Fresh chives, for garnish

Instructions:

1. In a large pot, heat the olive oil over medium heat. Add the chopped leeks and sauté until softened, about 5 minutes.

2. Add the chopped cauliflower to the pot and sauté for another 5 minutes.

3. Pour in the vegetable broth and bring the soup to a boil. Reduce the heat to low and simmer for 15-20 minutes, or until the cauliflower is tender.

4. Use an immersion blender to puree the soup until smooth. Alternatively, transfer the soup to a blender and blend until smooth, then return it to the pot.

5. Stir in the almond milk until well combined. Simmer for another 5 minutes.

6. Season the soup with salt and pepper to taste. Serve hot, garnished with fresh chives.

Cooking Time: 30 minutes
Serving Size: 4 servings

Pro Tip: For added flavor, you can stir in some grated Parmesan cheese or a sprinkle of nutmeg before serving.

White Bean and Kale Soup:

Ingredients:

- 1 tablespoon olive oil
- 1 onion, chopped
- 2 cloves garlic, minced
- 2 carrots, diced
- 2 celery stalks, diced
- 2 cups chopped kale
- 2 cans (15 ounces each) white beans, drained and rinsed
- 4 cups low-sodium vegetable broth
- 1 teaspoon dried thyme
- Salt and pepper, to taste
- Fresh lemon wedges, for serving

Instructions:

1. In a large pot, heat the olive oil over medium heat. Add the chopped onion and sauté until softened, about 5 minutes.
2. Add the minced garlic, diced carrots, and diced celery to the pot and sauté for another 5 minutes.
3. Stir in the chopped kale and sauté until wilted, about 2-3 minutes.
4. Add the drained and rinsed white beans, vegetable broth, and dried thyme to the pot. Bring to a boil, then reduce the heat to low and simmer for 15-20 minutes.
5. Season the soup with salt and pepper to taste. Serve hot, with fresh lemon wedges for squeezing over each bowl before eating.

Cooking Time: 30 minutes
Serving Size: 4 servings

Pro Tip: For added richness and creaminess, you can stir in a splash of coconut milk or heavy cream before serving.

Spinach and Chickpea Soup:

Ingredients:

- 1 tablespoon olive oil
- 1 onion, chopped
- 2 cloves garlic, minced
- 1 teaspoon ground cumin
- 1/2 teaspoon ground coriander
- 1/4 teaspoon ground cinnamon
- 4 cups low-sodium vegetable broth
- 1 can (15 ounces) chickpeas, drained and rinsed
- 4 cups chopped spinach
- Salt and pepper, to taste
- Greek yogurt, for garnish (optional)

Instructions:

1. In a large pot, heat the olive oil over medium heat. Add the chopped onion and sauté until softened, about 5 minutes.
2. Add the minced garlic, ground cumin, ground coriander, and ground cinnamon to the pot. Sauté for another minute, until fragrant.
3. Pour in the vegetable broth and bring the soup to a boil. Reduce the heat to low and simmer for 10 minutes.
4. Add the drained and rinsed chickpeas and chopped spinach to the pot. Simmer for another 5 minutes, or until the spinach is wilted.
5. Season the soup with salt and pepper to taste. Serve hot, with a dollop of Greek yogurt on top if desired.

Cooking Time: 20 minutes
Serving Size: 4 servings

Pro Tip: For added richness and creaminess, you can stir in a splash of coconut milk or heavy cream before serving.

Potato Leek Soup (low-fat version):

Ingredients:

- 1 tablespoon olive oil
- 2 leeks, white and light green parts only, chopped
- 2 cloves garlic, minced
- 2 potatoes, peeled and diced
- 4 cups low-sodium vegetable broth
- 1 cup unsweetened almond milk
- Salt and pepper, to taste
- Fresh chives, for garnish

Instructions:

1. In a large pot, heat the olive oil over medium heat. Add the chopped leeks and sauté until softened, about 5 minutes.
2. Add the minced garlic to the pot and sauté for another minute, until fragrant.
3. Add the diced potatoes and vegetable broth to the pot. Bring to a boil, then reduce the heat to low and simmer for 15-20 minutes, or until the potatoes are tender.
4. Use an immersion blender to partially puree the soup, leaving some chunks of potato for texture. Alternatively, transfer half of the soup to a blender and

blend until smooth, then return it to the pot.

5. Stir in the almond milk until well combined. Simmer for another 5 minutes.
6. Season the soup with salt and pepper to taste. Serve hot, garnished with fresh chives.

Cooking Time: 30 minutes
Serving Size: 4 servings

Pro Tip: For added flavor, you can stir in some chopped cooked bacon or ham before serving.

Turmeric Chicken Soup with Spinach:

Ingredients:

- 1 tablespoon olive oil
- 1 onion, chopped
- 2 cloves garlic, minced
- 1 teaspoon ground turmeric
- 6 cups low-sodium chicken broth
- 2 cups cooked chicken, shredded or diced
- 4 cups chopped spinach
- Juice of 1 lemon
- Salt and pepper, to taste
- Fresh cilantro, for garnish

Instructions:

1. In a large pot, heat the olive oil over medium heat. Add the chopped onion and sauté until softened, about 5 minutes.
2. Add the minced garlic and ground turmeric to the pot and sauté for another minute, until fragrant.
3. Pour in the chicken broth and bring the soup to a boil. Reduce the heat to low and simmer for 10 minutes.
4. Add the cooked chicken and chopped spinach to the pot. Simmer for another 5 minutes, or until the spinach is wilted.
5. Stir in the lemon juice and season the soup with salt and pepper to taste.
6. Ladle the soup into bowls and garnish with fresh cilantro before serving.

Cooking Time: 20 minutes
Serving Size: 4 servings

Pro Tip: For added warmth and spice, you can add a pinch of red pepper flakes or a dash of cayenne pepper to the soup before serving.

Creamy Broccoli Soup:

Ingredients:

- 1 tablespoon olive oil
- 1 onion, chopped
- 2 cloves garlic, minced
- 1 head broccoli, chopped
- 4 cups low-sodium vegetable broth
- 1/2 cup unsweetened almond milk
- 1/4 cup nutritional yeast (optional, for added flavor)
- Salt and pepper, to taste
- Toasted almond slices, for garnish

Instructions:

1. In a large pot, heat the olive oil over medium heat. Add the chopped onion and garlic, and sauté until softened, about 5 minutes.
2. Add the chopped broccoli to the pot and sauté for another 5 minutes.
3. Pour in the vegetable broth and bring the soup to a boil. Reduce the heat to low and simmer for 10-15 minutes, or until the broccoli is tender.
4. Use an immersion blender to puree the soup until smooth. Alternatively, transfer the soup to a blender and blend until smooth, then return it to the pot.
5. Stir in the almond milk and nutritional yeast (if using) until well combined. Simmer for another 5 minutes.
6. Season the soup with salt and pepper to taste. Serve hot, garnished with toasted almond slices.

Cooking Time: 30 minutes
Serving Size: 4 servings

Pro Tip: For added richness, you can stir in a splash of coconut milk or heavy cream before serving.

Tomato Lentil Soup:

Ingredients:

- 1 tablespoon olive oil
- 1 onion, chopped
- 2 cloves garlic, minced
- 1 carrot, diced
- 1 celery stalk, diced
- 1 cup dried red lentils, rinsed
- 1 can (14 ounces) diced tomatoes
- 4 cups low-sodium vegetable broth
- 1 teaspoon dried thyme

- Salt and pepper, to taste
- Fresh parsley, for garnish

Instructions:

1. In a large pot, heat the olive oil over medium heat. Add the chopped onion, garlic, carrot, and celery, and sauté until softened, about 5 minutes.
2. Add the rinsed red lentils, diced tomatoes (with their juices), vegetable broth, and dried thyme to the pot. Bring to a boil, then reduce the heat to low and simmer for 20-25 minutes, or until the lentils are tender.
3. Season the soup with salt and pepper to taste. Serve hot, garnished with fresh parsley.

Cooking Time: 30 minutes
Serving Size: 4 servings

Pro Tip: For added richness and creaminess, you can stir in a splash of coconut milk or heavy cream before serving.

Chicken and Rice Soup:

Ingredients:

- 1 tablespoon olive oil
- 1 onion, chopped
- 2 cloves garlic, minced
- 2 carrots, diced
- 2 celery stalks, diced
- 6 cups low-sodium chicken broth
- 1 cup cooked chicken, shredded or diced
- 1/2 cup uncooked white rice
- 1 teaspoon dried thyme
- Salt and pepper, to taste
- Fresh parsley, for garnish

Instructions:

1. In a large pot, heat the olive oil over medium heat. Add the chopped onion, garlic, carrot, and celery, and sauté until softened, about 5 minutes.
2. Pour in the chicken broth and bring the soup to a boil. Reduce the heat to low and simmer for 10 minutes.
3. Add the cooked chicken, uncooked white rice, and dried thyme to the pot. Simmer for another 15-20 minutes, or until the rice is cooked and tender.

4. Season the soup with salt and pepper to taste. Serve hot, garnished with fresh parsley.

Cooking Time: 30 minutes
Serving Size: 4 servings

Pro Tip: For added flavor, you can stir in some freshly grated Parmesan cheese or a squeeze of lemon juice before serving.

Coconut Curry Chicken Soup:

Ingredients:

- 1 tablespoon olive oil
- 1 onion, chopped
- 2 cloves garlic, minced
- 1 tablespoon curry powder
- 6 cups low-sodium chicken broth
- 1 can (14 ounces) coconut milk
- 2 cups cooked chicken, shredded or diced
- 1 red bell pepper, thinly sliced
- 1 cup chopped spinach or kale
- Salt and pepper, to taste
- Fresh cilantro, for garnish

Instructions:

1. In a large pot, heat the olive oil over medium heat. Add the chopped onion and sauté until softened, about 5 minutes.
2. Add the minced garlic and curry powder to the pot and sauté for another minute, until fragrant.
3. Pour in the chicken broth and coconut milk, and bring the soup to a boil. Reduce the heat to low and simmer for 10 minutes.
4. Add the cooked chicken, sliced red bell pepper, and chopped spinach or kale to the pot. Simmer for another 5 minutes, or until the vegetables are tender.
5. Season the soup with salt and pepper to taste. Serve hot, garnished with fresh cilantro.

Cooking Time: 25 minutes
Serving Size: 4 servings

Pro Tip: For added heat, you can add a pinch of red pepper flakes or a drizzle of sriracha sauce to the soup before serving.

Whole Grain Variation

Quinoa Salad with Roasted Vegetables

Ingredients:
- Cooked quinoa
- Bell peppers
- Zucchini
- Cherry tomatoes
- Lemon-tahini dressing (made with lemon juice, tahini, olive oil, garlic, salt, and pepper)

Instructions:
1. Preheat the oven to 400°F (200°C).
2. Chop the bell peppers and zucchini into bite-sized pieces.
3. Place the chopped vegetables on a baking sheet lined with parchment paper
4. Roast in the preheated oven for 20-25 minutes or until tender and slightly caramelized.
5. In a large bowl, combine the cooked quinoa and roasted vegetables.
6. Drizzle with lemon-tahini dressing and toss to coat.

Cooking Time: 30-35 minutes
Serving Size: 4

Pro Tip: Customize your salad with additional toppings such as crumbled feta cheese, toasted nuts, or fresh herbs like parsley or basil.

Brown Rice Buddha Bowl

Ingredients:
- Cooked brown rice
- Broccoli
- Avocado
- Shredded carrots
- Edamame
- Sesame seeds
- Miso dressing (made with miso paste, rice vinegar, soy sauce, sesame oil, and honey)

Instructions:
1. Steam the broccoli until tender-crisp.
2. Assemble bowls with cooked brown rice as the base.
3. Top with steamed broccoli, sliced avocado, shredded carrots, and edamame.
4. Sprinkle with sesame seeds.
5. Drizzle with miso dressing.

Cooking Time: 20 minutes
Serving Size: 2

Pro Tip: Add a protein boost by including grilled tofu or tempeh in your Buddha bowl.

Whole Wheat Pasta Primavera

Ingredients:
- Whole wheat pasta
- Spinach
- Cherry tomatoes
- Asparagus
- Olive oil
- Parmesan cheese

Instructions:

1. Cook the whole wheat pasta according to package instructions until al dente.
2. In a separate pan, sauté spinach, halved cherry tomatoes, and chopped asparagus until tender.
3. Drain the pasta and toss with the sautéed vegetables.
4. Drizzle with olive oil and sprinkle with Parmesan cheese.

Cooking Time: 15 minutes
Serving Size: 4

Pro Tip: For added protein, toss in cooked shrimp or grilled chicken breast.

Barley and Vegetable Soup

Ingredients:
- Barley
- Vegetable broth
- Carrots
- Celery
- Onion
- Fresh thyme
- Fresh parsley

Instructions:

1. In a large pot, bring vegetable broth to a boil.
2. Add barley and reduce heat to simmer. Cook until barley is tender, about 45-50 minutes.
3. Meanwhile, chop carrots, celery, and onions.
4. Add chopped vegetables to the pot with barley and continue to simmer until vegetables are tender, about 15-20 minutes.
5. Season with fresh thyme and parsley before serving.

Cooking Time: 1 hour 15 minutes
Serving Size: 6

Pro Tip: Make a large batch and freeze individual portions for quick and easy lunches throughout the week.

Farro and Chickpea Salad

Ingredients:
- Farro
- Chickpeas
- Cucumber
- Cherry tomatoes
- Fresh parsley
- Olive oil
- Lemon juice
- Garlic

Instructions:
1. Cook farro according to package instructions until tender.
2. Rinse and drain chickpeas.
3. Chop cucumber and halve cherry tomatoes.
4. In a large bowl, combine cooked farro, chickpeas, cucumber, cherry tomatoes, and chopped parsley.
5. Dress with olive oil, lemon juice, and minced garlic.

Cooking Time: 30 minutes
Serving Size: 4

Pro Tip: Add crumbled feta cheese or diced avocado for extra creaminess and flavor.

Buckwheat Stir-Fry

Ingredients:
- Buckwheat groats
- Bell peppers
- Snap peas
- Mushrooms
- Low-sodium soy sauce
- Sesame seeds

Instructions:
1. Heat a tablespoon of oil in a skillet over medium heat.
2. Add cooked buckwheat groats and stir-fry for 3-4 minutes.
3. Add sliced bell peppers, snap peas, and sliced mushrooms. Stir-fry until vegetables are tender-crisp.
4. Drizzle with low-sodium soy sauce and sprinkle with sesame seeds before serving.

Cooking Time: 20 minutes
Serving Size: 3
Pro Tip: For a protein boost, add diced tofu or cooked shrimp to the stir-fry.

Quinoa Stuffed Bell Peppers

Ingredients:

- Bell peppers
- Cooked quinoa
- Black beans
- Corn
- Diced tomatoes
- Fresh cilantro

Instructions:

1. Preheat the oven to 375°F (190°C).
2. Cut bell peppers in half and remove seeds and membranes.
3. In a bowl, mix cooked quinoa, black beans, corn, diced tomatoes, and chopped cilantro.
4. Stuff the bell pepper halves with the quinoa mixture.
5. Place stuffed peppers in a baking dish and bake for 25-30 minutes until peppers are tender.

Cooking Time: 35-40 minutes
Serving Size: 4 (2 halves per serving)

Pro Tip: Top stuffed peppers with shredded cheese during the last 5 minutes of baking for extra indulgence.

Spelt Salad with Grilled Vegetables

Ingredients:

- Spelt grains
- Eggplant
- Zucchini
- Red onion
- Fresh basil
- Balsamic vinaigrette (made with balsamic vinegar, olive oil, Dijon mustard, honey, garlic, salt, and pepper)

Instructions:

1. Cook spelt grains according to package instructions until tender.
2. Preheat the grill or grill pan to medium-high heat.
3. Slice eggplant, zucchini, and red onion into rounds.
4. Grill vegetables until tender and slightly charred, about 3-4 minutes per side.
5. In a large bowl, toss cooked spelt grains with grilled vegetables and chopped fresh basil.
6. Drizzle with balsamic vinaigrette and toss to coat.

Cooking Time: 25 minutes
Serving Size: 4

Pro Tip: Allow grilled vegetables to cool slightly before tossing with spelt grains to prevent wilting.

Millet Pilaf with Roasted Root Vegetables

Ingredients:
- Millet
- Carrots
- Parsnips
- Sweet potatoes
- Olive oil
- Fresh thyme
- Fresh rosemary

Instructions:
1. Cook millet according to package instructions until fluffy.
2. Preheat the oven to 400°F (200°C).
3. Peel and dice carrots, parsnips, and sweet potatoes.
4. Toss diced vegetables with olive oil, fresh thyme, and fresh rosemary.
5. Spread vegetables in a single layer on a baking sheet and roast for 25-30 minutes until caramelized and tender.
6. Serve roasted vegetables over cooked millet pilaf.

Cooking Time: *45-50 minutes*
Serving Size: *4*

Pro Tip: Add a handful of toasted nuts or seeds for extra crunch and flavor.

Whole Grain Wrap with Hummus and Veggies

Ingredients:
- Whole grain wraps
- Hummus
- Cucumber
- Lettuce
- Carrots
- Avocado

Instructions:
1. Spread a generous layer of hummus evenly over each whole grain wrap.
2. Thinly slice cucumber and avocado.
3. Shred lettuce and grate carrots.
4. Layer cucumber, lettuce, carrots, and avocado slices on top of the hummus.
5. Roll up tightly and slice into pinwheels for a portable lunch option.

Cooking Time: *None*
Serving Size: *2 wraps*

Pro Tip: Wrap pinwheels tightly in plastic wrap or foil to prevent them from falling apart when transporting them for lunch.

Chapter 4

Evening Serenity: Dinner Solutions

As the day winds down and the evening beckons, it's time to settle in for a comforting meal that nourishes both body and soul. In this chapter, we'll guide you through a collection of flavorful and soothing dinner options specifically crafted to alleviate the discomfort of acid reflux while tantalizing your taste buds. Let's start by banishing the misconception that reflux-friendly dinners are synonymous with bland and boring. On the contrary, our recipes are bursting with vibrant flavors and wholesome ingredients that will leave you feeling satisfied and content.

Picture this: a steaming bowl of aromatic chicken soup, infused with herbs and spices that not only warm the body but also soothe the stomach. Or perhaps a hearty turkey meatloaf, oozing with savory goodness and served alongside a medley of roasted vegetables, creating a symphony of flavors that dance on your palate.

But wait, there's more! How about a succulent salmon filet, delicately seasoned and baked to perfection, paired with a side of fluffy quinoa and sautéed greens? This dish not only satisfies your cravings for something substantial but also provides a nutritious and reflux-friendly option that won't leave you feeling heavy or uncomfortable. And let's not forget about the classics with a twist. Take our light and zesty shrimp stir-fry, for example. Bursting with colorful veggies and tossed in a tangy sauce, this dish proves that you can enjoy your favorite Asian-inspired flavors without worrying about the repercussions of acid reflux.

Of course, no dinner is complete without a sweet treat to round off the meal. Indulge in our guilt-free dessert options, from refreshing fruit salads to decadent yogurt parfaits, each offering a satisfyingly sweet ending to your evening without the fear of triggering reflux symptoms.

So, whether you're cooking for yourself, your family, or your friends, rest assured that our dinner solutions will not only satisfy your cravings but also support your journey towards digestive wellness. Say goodbye to dinnertime dilemmas and hello to evenings filled with serenity and satisfaction, one delicious dish at a time.

Herbs and Spices Soup

Chicken and Rice Soup with Fresh Thyme:

Ingredients:

- 1 tablespoon olive oil
- 1 onion, diced
- 2 carrots, sliced
- 2 celery stalks, sliced
- 1-pound boneless, skinless chicken breasts, diced
- 6 cups chicken broth
- 1 cup cooked rice
- 2 tablespoons fresh thyme leaves
- Salt and pepper to taste

Instructions:

1. In a large pot, heat olive oil over medium heat. Add diced onion, carrots, and celery, and cook until softened, about 5 minutes.
2. Add diced chicken breasts to the pot and cook until browned on all sides.
3. Pour in chicken broth and bring to a simmer. Cook for 15-20 minutes, until chicken is cooked through.
4. Stir in cooked rice and fresh thyme leaves. Season with salt and pepper, to taste.
5. Serve hot and enjoy the comforting flavors of this chicken and rice soup!

Cooking Time: 30-35 minutes
Serving Size: 4-6 servings

Pro Tips:

- For extra flavor, use homemade chicken broth or low-sodium chicken broth.
- Feel free to add additional vegetables, such as peas or corn, for extra nutrition.
- Garnish with fresh thyme leaves before serving for a beautiful presentation.

Turkey and Vegetable Soup with Rosemary:

Ingredients:

- 1 tablespoon olive oil
- 1 onion, diced
- 2 carrots, sliced

- 2 celery stalks, sliced
- 1 pound ground turkey
- 6 cups chicken or turkey broth
- 2 cups mixed vegetables (such as peas, corn, and green beans)
- 2 sprigs fresh rosemary
- Salt and pepper to taste

Instructions:

1. Heat olive oil in a large pot over medium heat. Add diced onion, carrots, and celery, and cook until softened, about 5 minutes.
2. Add ground turkey to the pot and cook until browned.
3. Pour in chicken or turkey broth and bring to a simmer. Add mixed vegetables and fresh rosemary sprigs.
4. Simmer for 20-25 minutes, until vegetables are tender and flavors have melded together.
5. Season with salt and pepper to taste before serving. Enjoy the hearty goodness of this turkey and vegetable soup!

Cooking Time: 35-40 minutes
Serving Size: 4-6 servings

Pro Tips:

- Use leftover cooked turkey or rotisserie chicken for a convenient shortcut.
- Substitute barley with brown rice or quinoa for a gluten-free option.
- Garnish with fresh rosemary leaves for an aromatic touch.

Beef and Barley Soup with Parsley:

Ingredients:

- 1 tablespoon olive oil
- 1 onion, diced
- 2 carrots, sliced
- 2 celery stalks, sliced
- 1 pound beef stew meat, cubed
- 6 cups beef broth
- 1/2 cup pearl barley
- 2 tablespoons chopped fresh parsley
- Salt and pepper to taste

Instructions:

1. Heat olive oil in a large pot over medium heat. Add diced onion, carrots, and celery, and cook until softened, about 5 minutes.
2. Add cubed beef stew meat to the pot and cook until browned on all sides.
3. Pour in beef broth and bring to a simmer. Add pearl barley and

simmer for 45-50 minutes, until barley is tender.

4. Stir in chopped fresh parsley and season with salt and pepper to taste.

5. Ladle into bowls and serve piping hot. Enjoy the comforting flavors of this beef and barley soup!

Cooking Time: 60-65 minutes
Serving Size: 4-6 servings

Pro Tips:
- For added depth of flavor, brown the beef cubes before adding the broth.
- Use low-sodium beef broth to control the sodium content of the soup.
- This soup can be made ahead of time and stored in the refrigerator for up to 3 days, allowing the flavors to meld even further.

Lentil Soup with Cumin and Coriander:

Ingredients:

- 1 tablespoon olive oil
- 1 onion, diced
- 2 carrots, diced
- 2 celery stalks, diced
- 2 cloves garlic, minced
- 1 cup dried lentils, rinsed and drained
- 6 cups vegetable broth
- 1 teaspoon ground cumin
- 1 teaspoon ground coriander
- Salt and pepper to taste

Instructions:

1. Heat olive oil in a large pot over medium heat. Add diced onion, carrots, celery, and minced garlic, and cook until softened, about 5 minutes.
2. Add dried lentils to the pot and stir to combine with the vegetables.
3. Pour in vegetable broth and bring to a simmer. Add ground cumin and coriander, stirring to incorporate.
4. Simmer for 25-30 minutes, until the lentils are tender.
5. Season with salt and pepper to taste before serving. Enjoy the earthy flavors of this lentil soup with a hint of cumin and coriander!

Cooking Time: 35-40 minutes
Serving Size: 4-6 servings

Pro Tips:

- Feel free to add additional vegetables, such as spinach or kale for extra nutrition.
- For a thicker soup, blend a portion of the soup with an immersion blender before serving.
- Serve with a squeeze of fresh lemon juice for a burst of brightness.

Potato and Leek Soup with Chives:

Ingredients:

- 2 tablespoons butter
- 2 leeks, white and light green parts only, thinly sliced
- 4 potatoes, peeled and diced
- 4 cups vegetable broth
- 1/2 cup heavy cream
- 2 tablespoons of chopped fresh chives
- Salt and pepper to taste

Instructions:

1. In a large pot, melt butter over medium heat. Add sliced leeks and cook until softened, about 5 minutes.
2. Add diced potatoes to the pot and cook for another 5 minutes, stirring occasionally.
3. Pour in vegetable broth and bring to a simmer. Cook for 15-20 minutes, until potatoes are tender.
4. If using, stir in heavy cream for added creaminess.
5. Season with salt and pepper to taste, and sprinkle chopped fresh chives over the top before serving. Enjoy the comforting flavors of this potato and leek soup with a hint of chives!

Cooking Time: 30-35 minutes
Serving Size: 4-6 servings

Pro Tips:

- For a dairy-free option, substitute the heavy cream with full-fat coconut milk.
- Make sure to thoroughly clean the leeks, as they can often harbor dirt and grit between their layers.
- This soup can be made ahead of time and reheated before serving. Adjust the consistency with a little extra broth or water, if necessary.

Tomato Basil Soup with Oregano:

Ingredients:

- 2 tablespoons olive oil
- 1 onion, diced
- 2 cloves garlic, minced
- 2 cans (14 ounces each) diced tomatoes
- 4 cups vegetable broth
- 1/4 cup chopped fresh basil leaves
- 1 teaspoon dried oregano
- Salt and pepper to taste

Instructions:

1. Heat olive oil in a large pot over medium heat. Add diced onion and minced garlic, and cook until softened and fragrant, about 5 minutes.
2. Add diced tomatoes (with their juices) to the pot, along with vegetable broth.
3. Bring the mixture to a simmer and cook for 15-20 minutes to allow the flavors to meld.
4. Stir in chopped fresh basil and dried oregano, and season with salt and pepper to taste.
5. Use an immersion blender or transfer the soup to a blender in batches to puree until smooth.
6. Serve hot, garnished with additional fresh basil leaves if desired. Enjoy the comforting flavors of this tomato basil soup with a hint of oregano!

Cooking Time: 20-25 minutes
Serving Size: 4-6 servings

Pro Tips:

- For a smoother soup, use an immersion blender to puree the soup until smooth before adding the fresh basil.
- Adjust the thickness of the soup by adding more broth, if desired.
- Serve with a crusty bread or grilled cheese sandwich for a satisfying meal.

Carrot Ginger Soup with Turmeric:

Ingredients:

- 2 tablespoons olive oil
- 1 onion, diced
- 2 cloves garlic, minced
- 1 pound of peeled and chopped carrots
- 1-inch piece of fresh ginger, peeled and grated
- 4 cups vegetable broth

- 1 teaspoon ground turmeric
- Salt and pepper to taste
- Coconut milk or yogurt for serving (optional)

Instructions:

1. Heat olive oil in a large pot over medium heat. Add diced onion and minced garlic, and cook until softened and fragrant, about 5 minutes.
2. Add chopped carrots and grated ginger to the pot, and cook for another 5 minutes, stirring occasionally.
3. Pour in vegetable broth and bring to a simmer. Cook for 20-25 minutes, until carrots are tender.
4. Stir in ground turmeric, and season with salt and pepper to taste.
5. Use an immersion blender or transfer the soup to a blender in batches to puree until smooth.
6. Serve hot, with a swirl of coconut milk or yogurt if desired. Enjoy the vibrant flavors of this carrot ginger soup with a hint of turmeric!

Cooking Time: 25-30 minutes
Serving Size: 4-6 servings

Pro Tips:

- For extra creaminess, add a splash of coconut milk or heavy cream before serving.
- Adjust the consistency of the soup by adding more broth if needed.
- This soup can be made ahead of time and stored in the refrigerator for up to 3 days. Reheat gently on the stove before serving.

Butternut Squash Soup with Sage:

Ingredients:

- 2 tablespoons butter or olive oil
- 1 onion, diced;
- 2 cloves garlic, minced
- 1 butternut squash, peeled, seeded, and chopped
- 4 cups vegetable broth
- 1/2 teaspoon ground nutmeg
- 1/4 teaspoon ground cinnamon
- 1/4 cup chopped fresh sage leaves
- Salt and pepper to taste
- Heavy cream or coconut milk for serving (optional)

Instructions:

1. In a large pot, melt butter or heat olive oil over medium heat. Add diced onion and minced garlic, and cook until softened and fragrant, about 5 minutes.
2. Add chopped butternut squash to the pot, along with vegetable broth.
3. Bring the mixture to a simmer and cook for 20-25 minutes, until squash is tender.
4. Stir in ground nutmeg, ground cinnamon, and chopped fresh sage leaves, and season with salt and pepper to taste.
5. Use an immersion blender or transfer the soup to a blender in batches to puree until smooth.
6. Serve hot, with a drizzle of heavy cream or coconut milk if desired. Enjoy the cozy flavors of this butternut squash soup with a hint of sage!

Cooking Time: 30-35 minutes
Serving Size: 4-6 servings

Pro Tips:

- For extra richness, stir in a splash of heavy cream or coconut milk before serving.
- Toast the sage leaves in a dry skillet for a few seconds before garnishing the soup to enhance their flavor.
- This soup pairs wonderfully with crusty bread or a side salad for a complete meal.

Spinach and White Bean Soup with Garlic:

Ingredients:

- 2 tablespoons olive oil
- 1 onion, diced
- 2 cloves garlic, minced
- 4 cups vegetable broth
- 2 cans (15 ounces each) white beans, drained and rinsed
- 4 cups fresh spinach leaves
- 1 teaspoon dried thyme
- Salt and pepper to taste
- Grated Parmesan cheese for serving (optional)

Instructions:

1. Heat olive oil in a large pot over medium heat. Add diced onion and minced garlic, and cook until softened and fragrant, about 5 minutes.
2. Pour in vegetable broth and bring to a simmer. Add white

beans and dried thyme, stirring to combine.

3. Simmer for 10–15 minutes to allow the flavors to meld.
4. Stir in fresh spinach leaves and cook for an additional 5 minutes, until wilted.
5. Season with salt and pepper, to taste.
6. Serve hot, garnished with grated Parmesan cheese if desired. Enjoy the hearty flavors of this spinach and white bean soup with a hint of garlic!

Cooking Time: 20-25 minutes
Serving Size: 4-6 servings

Pro Tips:

- For added protein, stir in shredded cooked chicken or diced tofu before serving.
- Customize the soup by adding other vegetables such as diced carrots or celery.
- This soup can be easily doubled or tripled to feed a larger crowd or for meal prep purposes.

Mushroom and Wild Rice Soup with Thyme:

Ingredients:

- 2 tablespoons butter
- 1 onion, diced
- 2 cloves garlic, minced
- 8 ounces muslin mushrooms, sliced
- 1/2 cup wild rice
- 4 cups vegetable broth
- 2 tablespoons fresh thyme leaves
- Salt and pepper to taste

Instructions:

1. In a large pot, melt butter over medium heat. Add diced onion and minced garlic, and cook until softened and fragrant, about 5 minutes.
2. Add sliced mushrooms to the pot and cook until golden brown.
3. Stir in wild rice and vegetable broth, and bring to a simmer.
4. Cover and cook for 45-50 minutes, until rice is tender.
5. Stir in fresh thyme leaves, and season with salt and pepper to taste.
6. Serve hot, and enjoy the earthy flavors of this mushroom and wild rice soup with a hint of thyme!

Cooking Time: 55-60 minutes
Serving Size: 4-6 servings

Pro Tips:

- For added creaminess, stir in a splash of heavy cream or coconut milk before serving.
- Make sure to rinse the wild rice thoroughly before adding it to the soup to remove any excess starch.
- This soup reheats well and can be stored in the refrigerator for up to 3 days.

Cauliflower Soup with Paprika and Dill:

Ingredients:

- 2 tablespoons olive oil
- 1 onion, diced
- 2 cloves garlic, minced
- 1 head cauliflower, chopped
- 4 cups vegetable broth
- 1 teaspoon paprika
- 2 tablespoons chopped fresh dill
- Salt and pepper to taste

Instructions:

1. Heat olive oil in a large pot over medium heat. Add diced onion and minced garlic, and cook until softened and fragrant, about 5 minutes.
2. Add chopped cauliflower to the pot, along with vegetable broth.
3. Bring the mixture to a simmer and cook for 20-25 minutes, until cauliflower is tender.
4. Stir in paprika and chopped fresh dill, and season with salt and pepper to taste.
5. Use an immersion blender or transfer the soup to a blender in batches to puree until smooth.
6. Serve hot, and enjoy the comforting flavors of this cauliflower soup with a hint of paprika and dill!

Cooking Time: 30-35 minutes
Serving Size: 4-6 servings

Pro Tips:

- For extra richness, stir in a splash of heavy cream or coconut milk before serving.
- Garnish with a drizzle of olive oil and a sprinkle of smoked paprika for an extra flavor boost.
- This soup pairs well with crusty bread or a side salad for a complete meal.

Zucchini and Basil Soup with Mint

Ingredients:

- 2 tablespoons unsalted butter
- 1 onion, chopped
- 2 cloves garlic, minced
- 4 medium zucchinis, diced
- 4 cups vegetable broth
- 1/2 cup fresh basil leaves
- 2 tablespoons fresh mint leaves
- Salt and pepper to taste
- Lemon wedges for serving (optional)

Instructions:

1. In a large pot, melt the butter over medium heat. Add chopped onion and cook until softened, about 5 minutes.
2. Add minced garlic to the pot and cook for another minute until fragrant.
3. Add diced zucchini to the pot and sauté for 5 minutes.
4. Pour in vegetable broth and bring to a boil. Reduce heat and simmer for 15-20 minutes, or until zucchini is tender.
5. Stir in fresh basil leaves and fresh mint leaves. Cook for an additional 2 minutes.
6. Use an immersion blender to puree the soup until smooth. Alternatively, transfer the soup to a blender and blend until smooth, then return it to the pot.
7. Season with salt and pepper, to taste. Serve hot, with lemon wedges on the side for squeezing over the soup, if desired.

Cooking Time: 25-30 minutes
Serving Size: 4-6 servings

Pro Tips:

- For added creaminess, stir in a splash of heavy cream or coconut milk before serving.
- Garnish with additional fresh basil and mint leaves for a burst of flavor.
- This soup can be stored in the refrigerator for up to 3 days. Reheat gently on the stove before serving.

Broccoli and Cheddar Soup with Chives

Ingredients:

- 4 cups broccoli florets
- 1 onion, chopped
- 2 cloves garlic, minced
- 4 cups vegetable broth
- 1 cup shredded cheddar cheese

- 1/2 cup heavy cream
- Salt and pepper to taste
- Fresh chives for garnish

Instructions:

1. In a large pot, sauté the chopped onion and minced garlic until soft and fragrant.
2. Add the broccoli florets and vegetable broth to the pot. Bring to a simmer and cook until the broccoli is tender, about 15 minutes.
3. Using an immersion blender or regular blender, puree the soup until smooth.
4. Stir in the shredded cheddar cheese and heavy cream until they are melted and creamy.
5. Season with salt and pepper, to taste.
6. Ladle the soup into bowls and garnish with fresh chives before serving.

Cooking Time: Approximately 25 minutes
Serving Size: 4 servings

Pro Tips: For extra creaminess, blend half of the soup and leave the other half chunky before combining. Adjust the thickness of the soup by adding more or less vegetable broth, as desired.

Asparagus Soup with Lemon and Tarragon

Ingredients:

- 1 lb. asparagus, trimmed and cut into 1-inch pieces
- 1 onion, chopped
- 2 cloves garlic, minced
- 4 cups chicken or vegetable broth
- 1 lemon, zest and juice
- 2 tbsp. fresh tarragon, chopped
- Salt and pepper to taste
- Greek yogurt or sour cream for garnish (optional)

Instructions:

1. In a large pot, sauté the chopped onion and minced garlic until softened.
2. Add the asparagus pieces and chicken or vegetable broth to the pot. Bring to a boil, then reduce heat and simmer until the asparagus is tender, about 10 minutes.
3. Using an immersion blender or regular blender, puree the soup until smooth.
4. Stir in the lemon zest, lemon juice, and chopped tarragon. Season with salt and pepper, to taste.

5. Serve hot, garnished with a dollop of Greek yogurt or sour cream, if desired.

Cooking Time: Approximately 20 minutes
Serving Size: 4 servings

Pro Tips: Reserve a few asparagus tips for garnish to add texture to the soup. Adjust the tartness of the soup by adding more or less lemon juice according to your preference.

Sweet Potato and Coconut Soup with Curry

Ingredients:

- 2 large sweet potatoes, peeled and diced
- 1 onion, chopped
- 2 cloves garlic, minced
- 1 can (13.5 oz) coconut milk
- 4 cups vegetable broth
- 2 tbsp. curry powder
- Salt and pepper to taste
- Fresh cilantro for garnish

Instructions:

1. In a large pot, sauté the chopped onion and minced garlic until fragrant.
2. Add the diced sweet potatoes, coconut milk, vegetable broth, and curry powder to the pot. Bring to a boil, then reduce heat and simmer until the sweet potatoes are tender, about 20 minutes.
3. Using an immersion blender or regular blender, puree the soup until smooth.
4. Season with salt and pepper, to taste.
5. Ladle the soup into bowls and garnish with fresh cilantro before serving.

Cooking Time: Approximately 25 minutes
Serving Size: 4 servings

Pro Tips: For added creaminess, use full-fat coconut milk. Adjust the level of spiciness by adding more or less curry powder according to your taste preferences.

Red Lentil Soup with Cumin and Chili Powder

Ingredients:

- 1 cup red lentils, rinsed
- 1 onion, chopped
- 2 cloves garlic, minced

- 1 carrot, diced
- 1 can (14.5 oz) diced tomatoes
- 4 cups vegetable broth
- 1 tsp. ground cumin
- 1/2 teaspoon chili powder
- Salt and pepper to taste
- Fresh cilantro for garnish

Instructions:

1. In a large pot, sauté the chopped onion and minced garlic vegetables.
2. Add the diced carrot, rinsed red lentils, diced tomatoes (with juices), vegetables until peppers, cumin, and chili powder to the pot. Bring to a boil, then reduce heat and simmer until peppers are cooked through and tender, about 20 minutes.
3. Season with salt and pepper, to taste.
4. Serve hot, garnished with fresh cilantro leaves.

Cooking Time: Approximately 25 minutes
Serving Size: 4 servings

Pro Tips: For added texture, reserve some cooked lentils and stir them into the soup just before serving. pepper, and spice by adding more or less chili powder to suit your taste.

Stir-Fries and Protein

Chicken and Broccoli Stir-Fry with Brown Rice:

Ingredients:

- 1 lb. boneless, skinless chicken breast, thinly sliced
- 2 cups broccoli florets
- 2 cloves garlic, minced
- 1 tablespoon grated ginger
- 2 tablespoons low-sodium soy sauce
- 1 tablespoon sesame oil
- 2 cups cooked brown rice
- Salt and pepper to taste

Instructions:

1. Heat sesame oil in a large skillet over medium heat. Add minced garlic and grated ginger, and sauté for 1 minute.
2. Add sliced chicken breast to the skillet and cook until no longer pink, about 5-7 minutes.
3. Add broccoli florets to the skillet and cook until tender-crisp, about 3-4 minutes.
4. Stir in low-sodium soy sauce and cooked brown rice, tossing until well combined and heated through.
5. Season with salt and pepper, to taste.
6. Serve hot and enjoy!

Cooking Time: Approximately 20 minutes
Serving Size: 4 servings

Pro Tips:

- For extra flavor, marinate the chicken in the soy sauce and sesame oil mixture for 30 minutes before cooking.
- Feel free to add other vegetables, such as bell peppers or snap peas, for added nutrition and color.

Shrimp and Snow Pea Stir-Fry with Quinoa:

Ingredients:

- 1 lb. large shrimp, peeled and deveined
- 2 cups snow peas, trimmed
- 1 red bell pepper, sliced
- 2 cloves garlic, minced

- 1 tablespoon grated ginger
- 2 tablespoons low-sodium soy sauce
- 1 tablespoon rice vinegar
- 2 cups cooked quinoa
- 1 tablespoon olive oil
- Salt and pepper to taste

Instructions:

1. Heat olive oil in a large skillet over medium heat. Add minced garlic and grated ginger, and sauté for 1 minute.
2. Add shrimp to the skillet and cook until pink and opaque, about 2-3 minutes per side.
3. Add snow peas and sliced red bell pepper to the skillet and cook until vegetables are tender-crisp, about 3-4 minutes.
4. Stir in low-sodium soy sauce and rice vinegar, tossing until well combined.
5. Add cooked quinoa to the skillet and toss until heated through.
6. Season with salt and pepper, to taste.
7. Serve hot and enjoy!

Cooking Time: Approximately 15 minutes
Serving Size: 4 servings

Pro Tips:

- For a spicy kick, add a pinch of red pepper flakes to the stir-fry sauce.
- Garnish with chopped green onions or cilantro for added freshness and flavor.

Tofu and Bok Choy Stir-Fry with Buckwheat Noodles:

Ingredients:

- 14 oz. firm tofu, drained and cubed
- 2 bunches baby bok choy, chopped
- 1 red bell pepper, sliced
- 2 cloves garlic, minced
- 1 tablespoon grated ginger
- 3 tablespoons low-sodium soy sauce
- 1 tablespoon sesame oil
- 8 oz buckwheat noodles, cooked according to package instructions
- 1 tablespoon olive oil
- Salt and pepper to taste

Instructions:

1. Heat olive oil in a large skillet over medium heat. Add minced garlic

and grated ginger, and sauté for 1 minute.

2. Add cubed tofu to the skillet and cook until golden brown, about 4-5 minutes per side.

3. Add chopped bok choy and sliced red bell pepper to the skillet and cook until vegetables are tender, about 3-4 minutes.

4. In a small bowl, whisk together low-sodium soy sauce and sesame oil. Pour over the tofu and vegetables in the skillet, tossing until well coated.

5. Add cooked buckwheat noodles to the skillet and toss until heated through.

6. Season with salt and pepper, to taste.

7. Serve hot and enjoy!

Cooking Time: Approximately 20 minutes
Serving Size: 4 servings

Pro Tips:

- Pressing the tofu before cooking helps remove excess moisture and allows it to crisp up better.
- Feel free to add other vegetables, such as mushrooms or carrots, for added texture and flavor.

Beef and Asparagus Stir-Fry with Cauliflower Rice:

Ingredients:

- 1 lb. beef sirloin, thinly sliced
- 1 lb. asparagus, trimmed and cut into bite-sized pieces
- 1 onion, sliced
- 2 cloves garlic, minced
- 1 tablespoon grated ginger
- 3 tablespoons low-sodium soy sauce
- 1 tablespoon rice vinegar
- 4 cups cauliflower rice
- 1 tablespoon olive oil
- Salt and pepper to taste

Instructions:

1. Heat olive oil in a large skillet over medium heat. Add minced garlic and grated ginger, and sauté for 1 minute.

2. Add sliced beef sirloin to the skillet and cook until browned, about 3-4 minutes per side.

3. Add trimmed asparagus and sliced onion to the skillet and cook until vegetables are tender-crisp, about 4-5 minutes.

4. In a small bowl, whisk together low-sodium soy sauce and rice vinegar. Pour over the beef and vegetables in the skillet, tossing until well coated.

5. Add cauliflower rice to the skillet and toss until heated through.

6. Season with salt and pepper, to taste.

7. Serve hot and enjoy!

Cooking Time: Approximately 20 minutes
Serving Size: 4 servings

Pro Tips:

- Choose lean cuts of beef like sirloin or flank steak to keep the dish lighter and more reflux-friendly.
- For added depth of flavor, sprinkle sesame seeds or chopped green onions on top before serving.

Salmon and Spinach Stir-Fry with Wild Rice:

Ingredients:

- 1 lb. salmon filet, cut into cubes
- 4 cups fresh spinach leaves
- 1 red bell pepper, sliced
- 2 cloves garlic, minced
- 1 tablespoon grated ginger
- 3 tablespoons low-sodium soy sauce
- 1 tablespoon honey
- 2 cups cooked wild rice
- 1 tablespoon olive oil
- Salt and pepper to taste

Instructions:

1. Heat olive oil in a large skillet over medium heat. Add minced garlic and grated ginger, and sauté for 1 minute.

2. Add cubed salmon filet to the skillet and cook until browned on all sides, about 4-5 minutes.

3. Add fresh spinach leaves and sliced red bell pepper to the skillet and cook until spinach is wilted and vegetables are tender, about 2-3 minutes.

4. In a small bowl, whisk together low-sodium soy sauce and honey. Pour over the salmon and vegetables in the skillet, tossing until well coated.

5. Add cooked wild rice to the skillet and toss until heated through.

6. Season with salt and pepper to taste.

7. Serve hot and enjoy!

Cooking Time: Approximately 15 minutes
Serving Size: 4 servings

Pro Tips:

- Opt for wild-caught salmon for its superior flavor and nutritional benefits.

- Feel free to substitute honey with maple syrup or agave nectar for a vegan-friendly option.

Turkey and Bell Pepper Stir-Fry with Barley:

Ingredients:

- 1 lb. ground turkey
- 2 bell peppers (any color), sliced
- 1 onion, sliced
- 2 cloves garlic, minced
- 1 tablespoon grated ginger
- 3 tablespoons low-sodium soy sauce
- 1 tablespoon rice vinegar
- 2 cups cooked barley
- 1 tablespoon olive oil
- Salt and pepper to taste

Instructions:

1. Heat olive oil in a large skillet over medium heat. Add minced garlic and grated ginger, and sauté for 1 minute.
2. Add ground turkey to the skillet and cook until browned, breaking it apart with a spoon, about 5-7 minutes.
3. Add sliced bell peppers and onion to the skillet and cook until vegetables are tender, about 3-4 minutes.
4. In a small bowl, whisk together low-sodium soy sauce and rice vinegar. Pour over the turkey and vegetables in the skillet, tossing until well coated.
5. Add cooked barley to the skillet and toss until heated through.
6. Season with salt and pepper, to taste.
7. Serve hot and enjoy!

Cooking Time: Approximately 20 minutes
Serving Size: 4 servings

Pro Tips:

- Use a mix of red, yellow, and green bell peppers for a colorful and visually appealing stir-fry.
- Substitute ground turkey with ground chicken or tofu for a lighter option.

Pork and Green Bean Stir-Fry with Forbidden Rice:

Ingredients:

- 1 lb. pork tenderloin, thinly sliced
- 2 cups green beans, trimmed and halved
- 1 carrot, julienned

- 2 cloves garlic, minced
- 1 tablespoon grated ginger
- 3 tablespoons low-sodium soy sauce
- 1 tablespoon hoisin sauce
- 2 cups cooked, forbidden rice
- 1 tablespoon sesame oil
- Salt and pepper to taste

Instructions:

1. Heat sesame oil in a large skillet over medium heat. Add minced garlic and grated ginger, and sauté for 1 minute.
2. Add thinly sliced pork tenderloin to the skillet and cook until browned and cooked through, about 4-5 minutes.
3. Add trimmed and halved green beans and julienned carrots to the skillet and cook until vegetables are tender-crisp, about 3-4 minutes.
4. In a small bowl, whisk together low-sodium soy sauce and hoisin sauce. Pour over the pork and vegetables in the skillet, tossing until well coated.
5. Add cooked forbidden rice to the skillet and toss until heated through.
6. Season with salt and pepper, to taste.
7. Serve hot and enjoy!

Cooking Time: Approximately 20 minutes,

Serving Size: 4 servings

Pro Tips:

- Marinate the pork slices in a mixture of soy sauce, garlic, and ginger for extra flavor before cooking.
- Forbidden rice, also known as black rice, is rich in antioxidants and adds a unique color and texture to the dish.

Tempeh and Brussels Sprout Stir-Fry with Millet:

Ingredients:

- 14 oz tempeh, cubed,
- 2 cups Brussels sprouts, trimmed and halved
- 1 red onion, sliced
- 2 cloves garlic, minced
- 1 tablespoon grated ginger
- 3 tablespoons low-sodium soy sauce
- 1 tablespoon maple syrup
- 2 cups cooked millet
- 1 tablespoon olive oil
- Salt and pepper to taste

Instructions:

1. Heat olive oil in a large skillet over medium heat. Add minced garlic and grated ginger, and sauté for 1 minute.
2. Add cubed tempeh to the skillet and cook until golden brown, about 4-5 minutes.
3. Add Brussels sprouts and sliced red onion to the skillet and cook until vegetables are tender, about 5-6 minutes.
4. In a small bowl, whisk together low-sodium soy sauce and maple syrup. Pour over the tempeh and vegetables in the skillet, tossing until well coated.
5. Add cooked millet to the skillet and toss until heated through.
6. Season with salt and pepper, to taste.
7. Serve hot and enjoy!

Cooking Time: Approximately 20 minutes
Serving Size: 4 servings

Pro Tips:

- Tempeh is a great source of plant-based protein and adds a hearty texture to the stir-fry.
- Feel free to substitute maple syrup with honey or agave nectar for a different flavor profile.

Chicken and Mushroom Stir-Fry with Jasmine Rice:

Ingredients:

- 1 lb. boneless, skinless chicken breast, thinly sliced
- 2 cups sliced mushrooms (any variety)
- 1 red bell pepper, sliced
- 2 cloves garlic, minced
- 1 tablespoon grated ginger
- 3 tablespoons low-sodium soy sauce
- 1 tablespoon rice vinegar
- 2 cups cooked jasmine rice
- 1 tablespoon sesame oil
- Salt and pepper to taste

Instructions:

1. Heat sesame oil in a large skillet over medium heat. Add minced garlic and grated ginger, and sauté for 1 minute.
2. Add thinly sliced chicken breast to the skillet and cook until no longer pink, about 5-7 minutes.
3. Add sliced mushrooms and sliced red bell pepper to the skillet and cook until vegetables are tender, about 4-5 minutes.

4. In a small bowl, whisk together low-sodium soy sauce and rice vinegar. Pour over the chicken and vegetables in the skillet, tossing until well coated.
5. Add cooked jasmine rice to the skillet and toss until heated through.
6. Season with salt and pepper, to taste.
7. Serve hot and enjoy!

Cooking Time: Approximately 20 minutes
Serving Size: 4 servings

Pro Tips:

- For extra flavor, marinate the chicken slices in the soy sauce and sesame oil mixture for 30 minutes before cooking.
- Use a mix of different mushroom varieties, such as shiitake, cremini, and oyster, for a more complex flavor profile.

Shrimp and Zucchini Stir-Fry with Couscous:

Ingredients:

- 1 lb. large shrimp, peeled and deveined
- 2 medium zucchinis, sliced
- 1 yellow bell pepper, sliced
- 2 cloves garlic, minced
- 1 tablespoon grated ginger
- 3 tablespoons low-sodium soy sauce
- 1 tablespoon honey
- 2 cups cooked couscous
- 1 tablespoon olive oil
- Salt and pepper to taste

Instructions:

1. Heat olive oil in a large skillet over medium heat. Add minced garlic and grated ginger, and sauté for 1 minute.
2. Add peeled and peppered shrimp to the skillet and cook until pink and opaque, about 2-3 minutes per side.
3. Add sliced zucchini and sliced yellow bell pepper to the skillet and cook until vegetables are tender-crisp, about 3-4 minutes.
4. In a small bowl, whisk together low-sodium soy sauce and honey. Pour over the shrimp and vegetables in the skillet, tossing until well coated.
5. Add cooked couscous to the skillet and toss until heated through.
6. Season with salt and pepper, to taste.
7. Serve hot and enjoy!

Cooking Time: Approximately 15 minutes
Serving Size: 4 servings

Pro Tips:

- To prevent overcooking, add the shrimp to the skillet only when the vegetables are nearly done.

- Garnish with freshly chopped parsley or cilantro for a burst of freshness and color.

Chapter 5

Satisfy Your Cravings: Wholesome Snacks for Between-Meal Treats

Are you tired of feeling hungry between meals but worried about triggering your acid reflux symptoms? Fear not! In this chapter, we're diving into the world of satisfying snacks that won't leave your stomach in knots. Say goodbye to the days of mindless munching on foods that aggravate your reflux, and hello to smart snacking solutions that nourish your body and soothe your stomach.

Let's face it—we all get those midday cravings that seem to strike out of nowhere. But instead of reaching for the nearest bag of chips or sugary snack, why not indulge in something that's not only delicious but also gentle on your digestive system? From crunchy veggies paired with creamy dips to protein-packed bites that keep you feeling full and satisfied, the options are endless when it comes to smart snacking.

Picture this: you're sitting at your desk, feeling that familiar pang of hunger creeping in. Instead of succumbing to the temptation of the office vending machine, you reach into your bag and pull out a container of crisp, colorful crudité and a small portion of hummus. With each crunchy bite, you feel refreshed and energized, knowing that you're nourishing your body without risking a reflux flare-up.

Or perhaps you're craving something a bit heartier to tide you over until dinner. In that case, why not whip up a batch of homemade energy balls? Packed with wholesome ingredients like oats, nuts, and dried fruit, these little bites of goodness are not only delicious but also easy to customize to your taste preferences. Plus, they're portable, making them the perfect on-the-go snack for busy days.

But snacking isn't just about satisfying hunger—it's also about treating yourself to something sweet every now and then. Luckily, you don't have to sacrifice your favorite indulgences just because you have acid reflux. With our collection of dessert-inspired snacks, you can satisfy your sweet tooth without the fear of discomfort. Thick creamy yogurt parfaits layered with fresh fruit and a sprinkle of granola, or frozen banana pops dipped in dark chocolate for a guilt-free treat that hits the spot every time.

So whether you're looking for something crunchy, creamy, or sweet, we've got you covered with a variety of satisfying snacks that are sure to keep your cravings at bay without aggravating your acid reflux. With a little creativity and some smart choices, you can snack your way to digestive comfort and peace of mind.

Snacks

Cucumber Rounds with Greek Yogurt and Dill:

Ingredients:
- Cucumber
- Greek yogurt
- Dill (fresh or dried)

Instructions:
1. Slice the cucumber into rounds.
2. Place a dollop of Greek yogurt on each cucumber round.
3. Sprinkle with dill to taste.

Almond Butter and Banana Rice Cakes:

Ingredients:
- Rice cakes
- Almond butter
- Banana

Instructions:
1. Spread almond butter onto each rice cake.
2. Top with sliced bananas.

Apple and Cheddar Cheese Slices:

Ingredients:
- Apple
- Cheddar cheese

Instructions:
1. Slice the apple into thin slices.
2. Place a small piece of cheddar cheese on each apple slice.

Hummus and Baby Carrots:

Ingredients:
- Baby carrots
- Hummus

Instructions:
1. Serve baby carrots with a side of hummus for dipping.

Avocado and Tomato Crackers:

Ingredients:
- Whole-grain crackers
- Avocado
- Cherry tomatoes

Instructions:

1. Spread mashed avocado onto each cracker.
2. Top with sliced cherry tomatoes.

Cream Cheese and Smoked Salmon Celery Sticks:

Ingredients:

- Celery sticks
- Cream cheese
- Smoked salmon

Instructions:

1. Fill each celery stick with cream cheese.
2. Top with a slice of smoked salmon.

Peaches and Honey Cottage Cheese:

Ingredients:

- Cottage cheese
- Peaches
- Honey

Instructions:

1. Mix diced peaches into cottage cheese.

2. Drizzle with honey to taste.

Seasoned Hard-Boiled Eggs:

Ingredients:

- Hard-boiled eggs
- Salt
- Pepper

Instructions:

1. Season hard-boiled eggs with a dash of salt and pepper.

Almond, Pumpkin Seed, and Cranberry Trail Mix:

Ingredients:

- Almonds
- Pumpkin seeds
- Dried cranberries

Instructions:

1. Mix almonds, pumpkin seeds, and dried cranberries together in a bowl.

Guacamole Dipped Bell Pepper Strips:

Ingredients:

- Bell peppers
- Guacamole

Instructions:

1. Slice bell peppers into strips.
2. Dip strips into guacamole.

Ricotta and Strawberry Toast:

Ingredients:

- Whole-grain bread
- Ricotta cheese
- Strawberries

Instructions:

1. Spread ricotta cheese onto toasted whole-grain bread.
2. Top with sliced strawberries.

Sea Salt Edamame Beans:

Ingredients:

- Edamame beans (cooked)
- Sea salt

Instructions:

1. Sprinkle cooked edamame beans with sea salt to taste.

Walnut-Served Sliced Pear:

Ingredients:

- Pear
- Walnuts

Instructions:

1. Slice the pear.
2. Serve with a handful of walnuts.

Nutritional Yeast and Garlic Powder Popcorn:

Ingredients:

- Popcorn kernels
- Nutritional yeast
- Garlic powder

Instructions:

1. Pop popcorn kernels.
2. Season with nutritional yeast and garlic powder to taste.

Tuna Salad Stuffed Mini Bell Peppers:

Ingredients:
- Mini bell peppers
- Tuna salad (pre-made)

Instructions:
1. Cut the tops off of mini bell peppers and remove seeds.
2. Stuff each pepper with tuna salad.

Oatmeal topped with sliced almonds and a drizzle of maple syrup:

Ingredients:
- Oatmeal
- Sliced almonds
- Maple syrup

Instructions:
1. Cook oatmeal according to package instructions.
2. Top with sliced almonds.
3. Drizzle with maple syrup.

Banana slices dipped in melted dark chocolate and frozen:

Ingredients:
- Bananas
- Dark chocolate (melted)

Instructions:
1. Slice bananas into rounds.
2. Dip each banana slice halfway into melted dark chocolate.
3. Place on a parchment-lined tray and freeze until chocolate is set.

Cottage cheese mixed with diced pineapple and a sprinkle of cinnamon:

Ingredients:
- Cottage cheese
- Diced pineapple
- Cinnamon

Instructions:
1. In a bowl, mix together cottage cheese and diced pineapple.
2. Sprinkle it with cinnamon before serving.

Whole grain pita chips served with tzatziki sauce for dipping:

Ingredients:
- Whole grain pita chips
- Tzatziki sauce

Instructions:
1. Serve whole grain pita chips with a side of tzatziki sauce for dipping.

Greek yogurt parfait layered with granola and mixed berries:

Ingredients:
- Greek yogurt
- Granola
- Mixed berries (such as strawberries, blueberries, raspberries)

Instructions:
1. In a glass or bowl, layer Greek yogurt, granola, and mixed berries.
2. Repeat layers as desired.

Steamed broccoli florets drizzled with lemon juice and olive oil:

Ingredients:
- Broccoli florets
- Lemon juice
- Olive oil

Instructions:
1. Steam broccoli florets until tender.
2. Drizzle with lemon juice and olive oil before serving.

Sliced kiwi paired with a small handful of cashews:

Ingredients:
- Kiwi
- Cashews

Instructions:
1. Slice kiwi into rounds.
2. Serve with a small handful of cashews.

Baked sweet potato fries seasoned with paprika and rosemary:

Ingredients:
- Sweet potatoes
- Paprika
- Rosemary

Instructions:
1. Cut sweet potatoes into fries.
2. Toss with paprika and rosemary.
3. Bake in the oven until crispy.

Cottage cheese topped with sliced peaches and a sprinkle of cinnamon:

Ingredients:
- Cottage cheese
- Sliced peaches
- Cinnamon

Instructions:
1. Top cottage cheese with sliced peaches.
2. Sprinkle it with cinnamon before serving.

Rice crackers spread with mashed avocado and sliced radishes:

Ingredients:
- Rice crackers
- Avocado
- Sliced radishes

Instructions:
1. Spread mashed avocado on rice crackers.
2. Top with sliced radishes.

Roasted chickpeas tossed in olive oil and cumin:

Ingredients:
- Chickpeas (canned or cooked)
- Olive oil
- Cumin

Instructions:
1. Toss chickpeas with olive oil and cumin.
2. Roast in the oven until crispy.

Cottage cheese mixed with diced mango and shredded coconut:

Ingredients:
- Cottage cheese
- Diced mango
- Shredded coconut

Instructions:
1. Mix cottage cheese with diced mango.
2. Sprinkle with shredded coconut before serving.

Steamed green beans served with a side of tahini sauce:

Ingredients:
- Green beans
- Tahini sauce

Instructions:
1. Steam green beans until tender.
2. Serve with a side of tahini sauce for dipping.

Whole grain tortilla chips served with salsa and sliced avocado:

Ingredients:
- Whole grain tortilla chips
- Salsa
- Sliced avocado

Instructions:
1. Serve whole grain tortilla chips with salsa and sliced avocado.

Frozen grapes served as a refreshing and sweet treat:

Ingredients:
- Grapes

Instructions:
1. Place grapes in the freezer until frozen.
2. Serve as a refreshing and sweet snack.

Chapter 6

Indulge Your Sweet Tooth: Dessert Delights

Are you ready to treat yourself to a world of sweet satisfaction without the discomfort of reflux? In this chapter, we're diving headfirst into a treasure trove of dessert recipes designed to tantalize your taste buds and soothe your stomach. From light and fruity to delightful rich, these sweet delights promise to be gentle on your digestion while delivering maximum flavor.

Let's start with a classic favorite: Fruit-Filled Crisps. Picture this—warm, juicy fruit topped with a crunchy, golden oat crumble. Whether it's a rustic apple crisp, a tangy berry medley, or a tropical twist with pineapple and coconut, these desserts are like a warm hug for your soul. But wait, there's more! How about a slice of creamy, dreamy cheesecake? Yes, you heard that right—cheesecake that won't send your reflux into overdrive. With a velvety smooth texture and a hint of tanginess, each bite is a decadent delight without the discomfort.

And let's not forget about everyone's favorite guilty pleasure: Chocolate! Indulge in a rich and velvety Chocolate Avocado Mousse, where ripe avocados lend their creamy texture to create a dessert that's as luxurious as it is satisfying. Or satisfy your chocolate cravings with a batch of Flourless Chocolate Brownies—dense, fudgy, and utterly irresistible. But perhaps you're craving something a little lighter? How about a refreshing lemon sorbet or a creamy coconut pudding? These desserts are perfect for those warm summer days when you want something sweet and refreshing without weighing you down.

And for those special occasions, why not whip up a batch of elegant Panna Cotta? With its delicate texture and subtle sweetness, it's sure to impress your guests while keeping your reflux at bay. No matter what your sweet tooth desires, these dessert delights offer a guilt-free way to indulge your cravings and satisfy your soul. So go ahead, treat yourself—you deserve it!

Light and Fruity

Mixed Berry Parfait:

Ingredients:
- Greek yogurt
- Fresh mixed berries (such as strawberries, blueberries, raspberries)
- Granola

Instructions:
1. In a glass or bowl, layer Greek yogurt, fresh mixed berries, and a sprinkle of granola.
2. Repeat the layers until the glass or bowl is filled.
3. Serve immediately for a refreshing and satisfying treat.

Watermelon Mint Salad:

Ingredients:
- Chunks of juicy watermelon
- Fresh mint leaves
- Lime juice

Instructions:
1. Toss chunks of watermelon with torn fresh mint leaves in a bowl.
2. Squeeze lime juice over the salad and toss gently to combine.
3. Serve immediately for a simple and hydrating dessert option.

Pineapple Coconut Sorbet:

Ingredients:
- Frozen pineapple chunks
- Coconut milk
- Lime juice

Instructions:
1. In a blender, combine frozen pineapple chunks, coconut milk, and lime juice.
2. Blend until smooth and creamy.
3. Transfer the mixture to a freezer-safe container and freeze until firm.
4. Scoop into bowls and serve for a creamy and tropical sorbet.

Citrus Salad with Honey-Lime Dressing:

Ingredients:
- Segments of oranges, grapefruits, and mandarins
- Honey
- Lime juice

Instructions:
1. Combine segments of oranges, grapefruits, and mandarins in a bowl.
2. In a small bowl, whisk together honey and lime juice to make the dressing.
3. Drizzle the dressing over the citrus salad and toss gently to coat.
4. Serve immediately for a zesty and vibrant dessert.

Strawberry Banana Smoothie Bowl:

Ingredients:
- Strawberries
- Bananas
- Almond milk
- Granola

Instructions:
1. In a blender, blend strawberries, bananas, and almond milk until smooth.
2. Pour the smoothie into a bowl.
3. Top with sliced bananas, strawberries, and a sprinkle of granola.
4. Serve immediately for a refreshing and crunchy smoothie bowl.

Mango Lime Popsicles:

Ingredients:
- Ripe mangoes
- Fresh lime juice
- Honey (optional)

Instructions:
1. In a blender, puree ripe mangoes with fresh lime juice and honey (if desired) until smooth.
2. Pour the mixture into popsicle molds.
3. Insert popsicle sticks and freeze until solid.
4. Once frozen, remove the popsicles from the molds and enjoy a refreshing and naturally sweet treat.

Grapefruit Granita:

Ingredients:
- Freshly squeezed grapefruit juice
- Mint leaves

Instructions:
1. Pour freshly squeezed grapefruit juice into a shallow pan.
2. Place the pan in the freezer and freeze until solid around the edges, about 1 hour.
3. Use a fork to scrape the frozen juice into icy flakes.
4. Serve immediately in bowls garnished with fresh mint leaves for a palate-cleansing dessert.

Berry Chia Seed Pudding:

Ingredients:
- Chia seeds
- Almond milk
- Maple syrup
- Fresh berries (such as strawberries, blueberries, raspberries)

Instructions:
1. In a jar or bowl, mix chia seeds with almond milk and maple syrup.
2. Stir well and let sit for 10 minutes to thicken.
3. Layer the chia seed pudding with fresh berries.
4. Serve chilled for a nutritious and satisfying pudding.

Peach Raspberry Cobbler:

Ingredients:
- Sliced peaches
- Raspberries
- Gluten-free oats
- Honey

Instructions:
1. Preheat the oven to 350°F (175°C).
2. In a baking dish, layer sliced peaches and raspberries.
3. In a separate bowl, mix gluten-free oats with honey to form a crumble topping.
4. Sprinkle the crumble topping over the fruit.
5. Bake for 30-35 minutes, or until the topping is golden brown and the fruit is bubbly.
6. Serve warm for a comforting dessert that won't trigger reflux.

Lemon Blueberry Frozen Yogurt:

Ingredients:
- Greek yogurt
- Fresh lemon zest
- Blueberries

Instructions:

1. In a bowl, mix Greek yogurt with fresh lemon zest and blueberries.
2. Transfer the mixture to a freezer-safe container.
3. Freeze until firm, about 4 hours.
4. Serve scoops of frozen yogurt for a tangy and refreshing dessert.

Rich and Delightful

Baked Apples with Cinnamon Oat Crumble

Ingredients:
- 4 large apples, cored
- 1/2 cup rolled oats
- 1/4 cup almond flour
- 2 tablespoons coconut oil, melted
- 2 tablespoons maple syrup
- 1 teaspoon ground cinnamon

Instructions:
1. Preheat the oven to 375°F (190°C).
2. Place the cored apples in a baking dish.
3. In a bowl, combine rolled oats, almond flour, melted coconut oil, maple syrup, and cinnamon to make the crumble topping.
4. Fill each apple with the oat crumble mixture.
5. Bake for 25-30 minutes or until the apples are tender and the topping is golden brown.
6. Serve warm and enjoy!

Greek Yogurt Parfait with Honey and Almonds

Ingredients:
- 1 cup Greek yogurt
- 2 tablespoons honey
- 2 tablespoons sliced almonds

Instructions:
1. In a glass or bowl, layer Greek yogurt, drizzle with honey, and sprinkle with sliced almonds.
2. Repeat layers as desired.
3. Serve immediately and enjoy the creamy, crunchy goodness!

Chia Seed Pudding with Mixed Berries

Ingredients:
- 1/4 cup chia seeds
- 1 cup almond milk
- 1 tablespoon honey or maple syrup (optional)
- 1 cup mixed berries (such as strawberries, blueberries, raspberries)

Instructions:

1. In a bowl, mix chia seeds and almond milk. If desired, sweeten with honey or maple syrup.
2. Let the mixture sit in the refrigerator for at least 2 hours or overnight to thicken.
3. Before serving, layer the chia seed pudding with mixed berries in glasses or bowls.
4. Enjoy the refreshing and nutrient-packed dessert!

Banana Bread Muffins with Walnuts

Ingredients:

- 2 ripe bananas, mashed
- 1/4 cup coconut oil, melted
- 1/4 cup maple syrup
- 1 teaspoon vanilla extract
- 1/2 cups almond flour
- 1/2 teaspoon baking soda
- 1/4 teaspoon salt
- 1/2 cup chopped walnuts

Instructions:

Preheat the oven to 350ºF (175ºC) and line a muffin tin with liners.

In a large bowl, mix mashed bananas, melted coconut oil, maple syrup, and vanilla extract.

1. Add almond flour, baking soda, and salt to the wet ingredients and mix until well combined.
2. Fold in chopped walnuts.
3. Divide the batter evenly among the muffin cups.
4. Bake for 20-25 minutes or until a toothpick inserted into the center comes out clean.
5. Let the muffins cool slightly before serving. Enjoy the moist and flavorful banana bread muffins!

Coconut Mango Rice Pudding

Ingredients:

- 1 cup cooked rice
- 1 cup coconut milk
- 1 ripe mango, diced
- 2 tablespoons maple syrup or honey
- 1/4 teaspoon vanilla extract
- Shredded coconut, for garnish (optional)

Instructions:

1. In a saucepan, combine cooked rice, coconut milk, diced mango, maple syrup or honey, and vanilla extract.

2. Cook over medium heat, stirring occasionally, until the mixture is heated through and thickened.
3. Remove from heat and let the pudding cool slightly.
4. Divide the rice pudding into serving bowls and garnish with shredded coconut, if desired.
5. Serve warm or chilled and savor the tropical flavors of coconut and mango!

Avocado Chocolate Mousse

Ingredients:
- 2 ripe avocados, peeled and pitted
- 1/4 cup cocoa powder
- 1/4 cup maple syrup or honey
- 1 teaspoon vanilla extract
- Pinch of salt

Instructions:
1. In a blender or food processor, combine ripe avocados, cocoa powder, maple syrup or honey, vanilla extract, and a pinch of salt.
2. Blend until smooth and creamy, scraping down the sides as needed.
3. Transfer the avocado chocolate mousse to serving dishes and chill in the refrigerator for at least 30 minutes before serving.
4. Garnish with fresh berries or shaved chocolate, if desired.
5. Enjoy the luscious and indulgent chocolate mousse made with the goodness of avocados!

Peach Cobbler with Almond Flour Crust

Ingredients:
- 4 cups sliced peaches
- 2 tablespoons maple syrup or honey
- 1 teaspoon vanilla extract
- 1 cup almond flour
- 1/4 cup coconut sugar
- 1/4 cup melted coconut oil
- 1/2 teaspoon ground cinnamon
- Pinch of salt

Instructions:
1. Preheat the oven to 350°F (175°C) and grease a baking dish.
2. In a bowl, toss sliced peaches with maple syrup or honey and vanilla extract.
3. Spread the peaches evenly in the prepared baking dish.
4. In another bowl, mix almond flour, coconut sugar, melted

coconut oil, ground cinnamon, and a pinch of salt until crumbly.

5. Sprinkle the almond flour mixture over the peaches.
6. Bake for 30-35 minutes or until the peaches are bubbly and the crust is golden brown.
7. Let the peach cobbler cool slightly before serving. Enjoy the comforting and flavorful dessert!

Lemon Blueberry Bars

Ingredients:
- 1 cup almond flour
- 1/4 cup coconut flour
- 1/4 cup coconut sugar
- 1/4 teaspoon baking soda
- Pinch of salt
- 1/4 cup coconut oil, melted
- 2 tablespoons lemon juice
- Zest of 1 lemon
- 1 egg
- 1 cup fresh blueberries
- Powdered sugar, for dusting (optional)

Instructions:
1. Preheat the oven to 350ºF (175ºC) and line a baking dish with parchment paper.
2. In a bowl, mix almond flour, coconut flour, coconut sugar, baking soda, and a pinch of salt.
3. Add melted coconut oil, lemon juice, lemon zest, and egg to the dry ingredients and mix until well combined.
4. Gently fold in fresh blueberries.
5. Press the mixture into the prepared baking dish and smooth the top with a spatula.
6. Bake for 20-25 minutes or until the edges are golden brown.
7. Let the lemon blueberry bars cool completely before cutting into squares.
8. Dust with powdered sugar, if desired, before serving. Enjoy the tangy and fruity dessert!

Raspberry Coconut Macaroons

Ingredients:
- 2 cups shredded coconut
- 1/4 cup coconut flour
- 1/4 cup coconut oil, melted
- 1/4 cup maple syrup or honey
- 1 teaspoon vanilla extract
- 1/2 cup fresh raspberries, chopped

Instructions:

- Preheat the oven to 325°F (160°C) and line a baking sheet with parchment paper.
- In a bowl, combine shredded coconut, coconut flour, melted coconut oil, maple syrup or honey, and vanilla extract.
- Fold in chopped raspberries until well incorporated.
- Scoop tablespoon-sized portions of the mixture and shape into macaroons using your hands.
- Place the macaroons on the prepared baking sheet and bake for 20-25 minutes or until golden brown.
- Let the raspberry coconut macaroons cool completely before serving. Enjoy the chewy and coconutty treats with bursts of raspberry flavor!

Chapter 7

Understanding the Importance of Meal Preparation and Beyond: A Key to Managing Acid Reflux

Meal prep isn't just about saving time—it's a powerful tool in the battle against acid reflux. Picture this: it's the end of a long day, your stomach is rumbling, and the last thing you want to do is spend hours in the kitchen trying to whip up a meal that won't leave you regretting it later. That's where meal prep comes in, swooping in like a superhero to save the day. But why is meal prep so important, especially when you're dealing with acid reflux? Let's break it down. When you're prepared with pre-planned meals and ingredients, you're less likely to reach for those quick-fix, convenience foods that are often loaded with reflux-triggering ingredients like spicy sauces or acidic marinades. Instead, you have a fridge stocked with wholesome, reflux-friendly options just waiting to be enjoyed.

Meal prep also takes the guesswork out of cooking, which can be a huge relief when you're dealing with the unpredictable nature of acid reflux. No more staring into the abyss of your pantry, wondering what on earth you can eat without setting off a reflux flare-up. With a well-thought-out meal plan in hand, you can approach cooking with confidence, knowing that each ingredient has been carefully chosen to support your digestive health. But perhaps the most important aspect of meal prep is the control it gives you over your diet. When you take the time to plan and prepare your meals ahead of time, you're less likely to find yourself in situations where you're forced to make hasty, reflux-triggering choices—like grabbing fast food on your lunch break or ordering takeout after a long day at work. Instead, you have the power to nourish your body with foods that support your health and well-being, all while keeping those pesky reflux symptoms at bay. So, how do you get started with meal prep? It's simpler than you might think. Start by carving out some time each week to plan your meals and grocery shop for the ingredients you'll need. Then, set aside a few hours to chop veggies, cook grains, and prepare proteins in advance. Invest in some quality storage containers to keep your prepped ingredients fresh throughout the week, and voila—you're ready to tackle even the busiest of days with ease.

In the end, meal prep isn't just about saving time or simplifying your life—it's about taking control of your health and well-being, one delicious meal at a time. So go ahead, embrace the power of meal prep, and watch as it transforms your relationship with food and your journey towards managing acid reflux.

4-Week Meal Plan

Week 1

Day	Breakfast	Lunch	Dinner	Snacks	Dessert	Smoothies
Mon	Tomato Basil Egg Cups	Spinach and Potato Soup	Beef and Asparagus Stir-Fry with Cauliflower Rice	Apple and Cheddar Cheese Slices	Watermelon Mint Salad	Pineapple Paradise
Tues	Tropical Oatmeal Delight	Mediterranean Chickpea Salad	Salmon and Spinach Stir-Fry with Wild Rice	Cream Cheese and Smoked Salmon Celery Sticks	Chia Seed Pudding with Mixed Berries	Kiwi Kiss
Wed	Spinach and Mushroom Omelet	Roasted Red Pepper Soup	Chicken and Rice Soup with Fresh Thyme	Avocado and Tomato Crackers	Greek Yogurt Parfait with Honey and Almonds	Blueberry Blast
Thurs	Carrot Cake Breakfast Cookies	Caprese Salad	Lentil Soup with Cumin and Coriander	Almond Butter and Banana Rice Cakes	Mixed Berry Parfait	Mango Tango
Fri	Broccoli and Cheese Quiche	Creamy Butternut Squash Soup	Turkey and Vegetable Soup with Rosemary	Peaches and Honey Cottage Cheese	Baked Apples with Cinnamon Oat Crumble	Banana Berry Bliss
Sat	Zucchini Fritters	Millet Pilaf with Roasted Root Vegetables	Chicken and Broccoli Stir-Fry with Brown Rice	Hummus and Baby Carrots	Citrus Salad with Honey-Lime Dressing	Peachy Keen
Sun	Classic Cinnamon Banana Oatmeal	Spelt Salad with Grilled Vegetables	Beef and Barley Soup with Parsley	Cucumber Rounds with Greek Yogurt and Dill	Pineapple Coconut Sorbet	Berry Banana Bonanza

Week 2

Day	Breakfast	Lunch	Dinner	Snacks	Dessert	Smoothies
Mon	Veggie Egg Scramble	Brown Rice Buddha Bowl	Turkey and Bell Pepper Stir-Fry with Barley	Walnut-Served Sliced Pear	Avocado Chocolate Mousse	Pineapple Banana Coconut Cream
Tues	Bell Pepper and Onion Frittata	Quinoa Salad with Roasted Vegetables	Tempeh and Brussels Sprout Stir-Fry with Millet	Ricotta and Strawberry Toast	Coconut Mango Rice Pudding	Grapefruit Granita
Wed	Blueberry Almond Flour Scones	Spinach and Strawberry Salad	Potato and Leek Soup with Chives	Oatmeal topped with sliced almonds and a drizzle of maple syrup	Lemon Blueberry Bars	Berry Chia Seed Pudding
Thurs	Mushroom and Swiss Cheese Frittata	Barley and Vegetable Soup	Chicken and Mushroom Stir-Fry with Jasmine Rice	Tuna Salad Stuffed Mini Bell Peppers	Grapefruit Granita	Mango Lime Popsicles
Fri	Banana Oat Muffins	Greek Salad	Carrot Ginger Soup with Turmeric	Nutritional Yeast and Garlic Powder Popcorn	Peach Cobbler with Almond Flour Crust	Citrus Salad with Honey-Lime Dressing
Sat	Almond Joy Oatmeal	Mixed Green Salad with Grilled Chicken	Tomato Basil Soup with Oregano	Banana slices dipped in melted dark chocolate and frozen	Lemon Blueberry Frozen Yogurt	Strawberry Banana Smoothie Bowl
Sun	Spinach and Feta Omelet	Whole Wheat Pasta Primavera	Pork and Green Bean Stir-Fry with Forbidden Rice	Sea Salt Edamame Beans	Banana Bread Muffins with Walnuts	Peach Raspberry Cobbler

Week 3

Day	Breakfast	Lunch	Dinner	Snacks	Dessert	Smoothies
Mon	Cauliflower Hash Browns	Coconut Cauliflower Soup	Tomato Basil Soup with Oregano	Steamed green beans served with a side of tahini sauce	Baked Apples with Cinnamon Oat Crumble	Berry Banana Bonanza
Tues	Ham and Swiss Breakfast Casserole	Turmeric Lentil Soup	Potato and Leek Soup with Chives	Whole grain pita chips served with tzatziki sauce for dipping	Lemon Blueberry Frozen Yogurt	Orange Creamsicle
Wed	Broccoli and Cheese Quiche	Fruit and Nut Salad	Tofu and Bok Choy Stir-Fry with Buckwheat Noodles	Banana slices dipped in melted dark chocolate and frozen	Pineapple Coconut Sorbet	Orange Carrot Concoction
Thurs	Southwest Egg Burritos	Spinach and Potato Soup	Mushroom and Wild Rice Soup with Thyme	Cottage cheese mixed with diced pineapple and a sprinkle of cinnamon	Watermelon Mint Salad	Pineapple Banana Coconut Cream
Fri	Smoked Salmon and Dill Egg Muffins	Panzanella Salad	Spinach and White Bean Soup with Garlic	Tuna Salad Stuffed Mini Bell Peppers	Raspberry Coconut Macaroons	Banana Berry Bliss
Sat	Tomato and Basil Frittata	Black Bean and Corn Salad	Cauliflower Soup with Paprika and Dill	Apple and Cheddar Cheese Slices	Lemon Blueberry Frozen Yogurt	Grapefruit Granita
Sun	Asparagus and Goat Cheese Omelet	Turmeric Lentil Soup	Lentil Soup with Cumin and Coriander	Greek yogurt parfait layered with granola and mixed berries	Peach Cobbler with Almond Flour Crust	Blueberry Blast

Week 4

Day	Breakfast	Lunch	Dinner	Snacks	Dessert	Smoothies
Mon	Tropical Oatmeal Delight	Caprese Salad	Tempeh and Brussels Sprout Stir-Fry with Millet	Nutritional Yeast and Garlic Powder Popcorn	Chia Seed Pudding with Mixed Berries	Berry Chia Seed Pudding
Tues	Carrot Cake Breakfast Cookies	Spelt Salad with Grilled Vegetables	Beef and Asparagus Stir-Fry with Cauliflower Rice	Greek yogurt parfait layered with granola and mixed berries	Peach Cobbler with Almond Flour Crust	Berry Banana Bonanza
Wed	Spinach and Feta Omelett	Roasted Red Pepper Soup	Chicken and Mushroom Stir-Fry with Jasmine Rice	Apple and Cheddar Cheese Slices	Avocado Chocolate Mousse	Blueberry Blast
Thurs	Cauliflower Hash Browns	Coconut Cauliflower Soup	Turkey and Bell Pepper Stir-Fry with Barley	Walnut-Served Sliced Pear	Pineapple Coconut Sorbet	Kiwi Kiss
Fri	Veggie Egg Scramble	Fruit and Nut Salad	Tomato Basil Soup with Oregano	Ricotta and Strawberry Toast	Citrus Salad with Honey-Lime Dressing	Peachy Keen
Sat	Classic Cinnamon Banana Oatmeal	Mediterranean Chickpea Salad	Potato and Leek Soup with Chives	Steamed green beans served with a side of tahini sauce	Watermelon Mint Salad	Pineapple Paradise
Sun	Tomato Basil Egg Cups	Brown Rice Buddha Bowl	Beef and Barley Soup with Parsley	Tuna Salad Stuffed Mini Bell Peppers	Lemon Blueberry Frozen Yogurt	Banana Berry Bliss

Conversion Table

Volume Measurements

1 tablespoon (tbsp)	=	15 milliliters (ml)
1 teaspoon (tsp)	=	5 milliliters (ml)
1 fluid ounce (fl oz)	=	30 milliliters (ml)
1 cup (c)	=	240 milliliters (ml)
1 pint (pt)	=	480 milliliters (ml)
1 quart (qt)	=	960 milliliters (ml)
1 gallon (gal)	=	3.8 liters (l)

Weight Measurements

1 ounce (oz)	=	28.35 grams (g)
1 pound (lb)	=	454 grams (g)
1 kilogram (kg)	=	1000 grams (g)

Common Ingredient Conversions

1 cup of flour	=	120 grams (g)
1 cup of sugar	=	200 grams (g)
1 cup of butter	=	227 grams (g)
1 cup of oats	=	90 grams (g)
1 cup of cooked quinoa	=	185 grams (g)
1 cup of cooked lentils	=	200 grams (g)
1 cup of cooked rice	=	185 grams (g)
1 cup of chopped vegetables	=	Approximately 150 grams (g)
1 medium-sized banana	=	Approximately 120 grams (g)
1 medium-sized avocado	=	Approximately 150 grams (g)
1 medium-sized tomato	=	Approximately 150 grams (g)
1 medium-sized chicken breast	=	Approximately 170 grams (g)
1 medium-sized salmon filet	=	Approximately 150 grams (g)
1 medium-sized beef steak	=	Approximately 200 grams (g)
1 medium-sized shrimp	=	Approximately 1 ounce (oz) or 28 grams (g)
1 medium-sized zucchini	=	Approximately 150 grams (g)
1 medium-sized bell pepper	=	Approximately 150 grams (g)
1 medium-sized onion	=	Approximately 150 grams (g)

Chapter 8

Cooking Challenge: The Acid Reflux Recipe Marathon

Welcome to the ultimate cooking challenge designed to put your culinary skills to the test while exploring a variety of delicious and reflux-friendly recipes. In this challenge, you'll embark on a journey through 30 days of flavorful dishes, each crafted to soothe your stomach and tantalize your taste buds. Are you ready to take on the Acid Reflux Recipe Marathon?

Challenge Rules:

1. Prepare one recipe from the provided list each day for 30 consecutive days.
2. Find each recipe group and class
3. Follow the recipe instructions carefully, ensuring accurate measurements and proper cooking techniques.
4. Share your cooking journey on social media using the hashtag #AcidRefluxChallenge to inspire others and document your progress.
5. Experiment with ingredient substitutions or variations to personalize each recipe to your taste preferences or dietary restrictions.
6. Stay consistent and committed to completing the challenge, embracing each cooking session as an opportunity to nourish your body and cultivate your culinary skills.

Challenge Recipes:

- Day 1: Veggie Egg Scramble
- Day 2: Brown Rice Buddha Bowl
- Day 3: Turkey and Bell Pepper Stir-Fry with Barley
- Day 4: Walnut-Served Sliced Pear

- Day 5: Avocado Chocolate Mousse
- Day 6: Pineapple Banana Coconut Cream
- Day 7: Bell Pepper and Onion Frittata
- Day 8: Quinoa Salad with Roasted Vegetables
- Day 9: Tempeh and Brussels Sprout Stir-Fry with Millet
- Day 10: Ricotta and Strawberry Toast
- Day 11: Coconut Mango Rice Pudding
- Day 12: Grapefruit Granita
- Day 13: Blueberry Almond Flour Scones
- Day 14: Spinach and Strawberry Salad
- Day 15: Potato and Leek Soup with Chives
- Day 16: Oatmeal topped with sliced almonds and a drizzle of maple syrup
- Day 17: Lemon Blueberry Bars
- Day 18: Berry Chia Seed Pudding
- Day 19: Mushroom and Swiss Cheese Frittata
- Day 20: Barley and Vegetable Soup
- Day 21: Chicken and Mushroom Stir-Fry with Jasmine Rice
- Day 22: Tuna Salad Stuffed Mini Bell Peppers
- Day 23: Grapefruit Granita
- Day 24: Mango Lime Popsicles
- Day 25: Banana Oat Muffins
- Day 26: Greek Salad
- Day 27: Carrot Ginger Soup with Turmeric
- Day 28: Nutritional Yeast and Garlic Powder Popcorn
- Day 29: Peach Cobbler with Almond Flour Crust
- Day 30: Citrus Salad with Honey-Lime Dressing

Get ready to embark on a culinary adventure filled with nourishing meals, creative flavors, and the satisfaction of conquering the Acid Reflux Recipe Marathon. Let's cook!

Recipe Journal

Recipe Journal

Recipe Journal

Recipe Journal

Recipe Journal

Recipe Journal

Recipe Journal

Recipe Journal

Recipe Journal

____
____
____
____
____
____
____
____
____
____
____
____
____

Recipe Journal

Recipe Journal

Recipe Journal

Recipe Journal

Recipe Journal

Recipe Journal

Recipe Journal

Recipe Journal

Recipe Journal

Recipe Journal